Pet owner educational atlas
SURGERY

All rights reserved.

No part of this book may be reproduced, stored or transmitted in any form or by any electronic or mechanical means, including photocopying or CD/DVD, without prior written permission from the publisher.

Any form of reproduction, distribution, publication or transformation of this book is only permitted with the authorisation of its copyright holders, apart from the exceptions allowed by law. Contact CEDRO (Spanish Centre of Reproduction Rights, www.cedro.org) if you need to photocopy or scan any part of this book (www.conlicencia.com; 91 702 19 70 / 93 272 04 47).

Warning:

Veterinary science is constantly evolving, as are pharmacology and the other sciences. Inevitably, it is therefore the responsibility of the veterinary clinician to determine and verify the dosage, the method of administration, the duration of treatment and any possible contraindications to the treatments given to each individual patient, based on his or her professional experience. Neither the publisher nor the author can be held liable for any damage or harm caused to people, animals or properties resulting from the correct or incorrect application of the information contained in this book.

This book has been published originally in Spanish under the title:
Atlas de información al propietario. Cirugía
© 2010 Grupo Asís Biomedia, S.L.
ISBN Spanish edition: 978-84-692-6914-5

For this English edition:
© 2014 Grupo Asís Biomedia, S.L.
Plaza Antonio Beltrán Martínez nº 1, planta 8 - letra I
(Centro empresarial El Trovador)
50002 Zaragoza - Spain

Translation:
Lexiapark, S.L.

Illustrators:
Jacob Gragera Artal
Juan Carlos Nuviala Ortín
Víctor Marco Cámara

Design and layout:
Servet editorial - Grupo Asís Biomedia, S.L.
www.grupoasis.com
info@grupoasis.com

Printing:
ULZAMA gráficas
Pol. Ind. Areta, calle A-35
31620 Huarte, Navarra

ISBN: 978-84-92569-39-7
D.L.: Z 939-2012

Printed in Spain

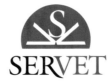

Contents

Preface

It is an indisputable fact that pet owners are increasingly demanding more from vets, expecting more detailed information on the conditions their pets are suffering from and clearer explanations of how we intend to solve their problems.

Graphic and audio-visual media have increasingly become our society's communication tools of choice. Verbal explanations accompanied by diagrams make it easier and quicker to transfer information and improve the successful understanding and assimilation of that information.

For a pet owner, the prospect of their pet undergoing an operation induces a degree of stress and anxiety. This atlas is a useful tool for explaining the nature of the pet's condition and the planned procedure, giving the pet owner greater understanding of and confidence in it, our work enabling them to make an informed choice.

This publication strikes the right balance between technical detail, with accurate anatomical and pathological features of various conditions, while still being accessible and engaging for the pet owner.

In addition, the material on which it is printed allows for annotations and sketches to be made and then easily erased so that it can be used time after time.

Finally, bond between the veterinarian and pet owner should be enhanced by clearer communication through the use of this book.

José Rodríguez Gómez
Veterinary surgeon

Pedicle skin flap

Illustration 1.1

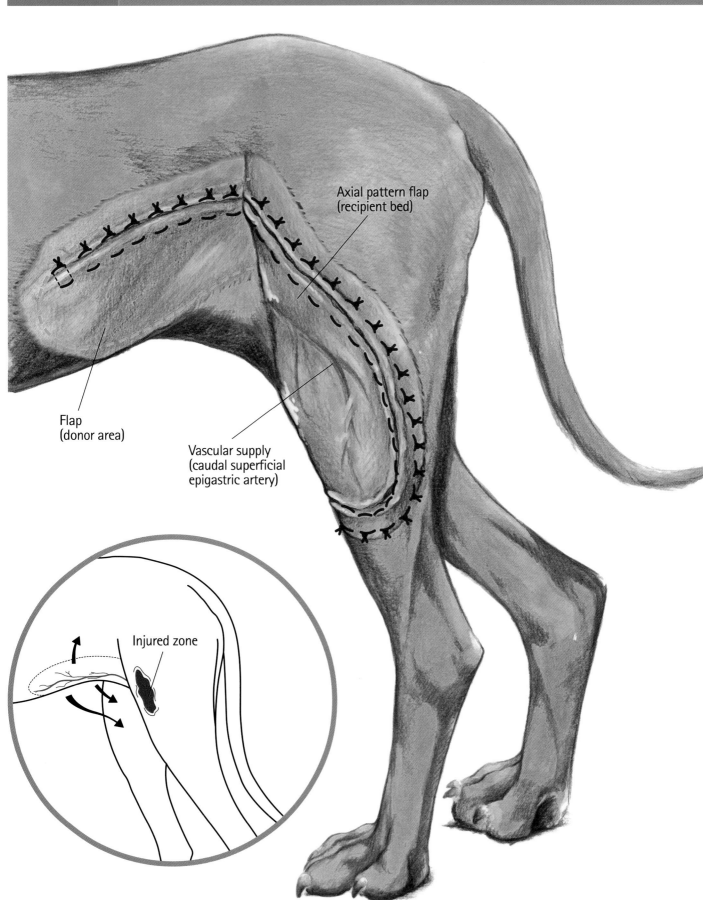

Axial pattern flap
(recipient bed)

Flap
(donor area)

Vascular supply
(caudal superficial
epigastric artery)

Injured zone

Mesh skin graft

Illustration 1.2

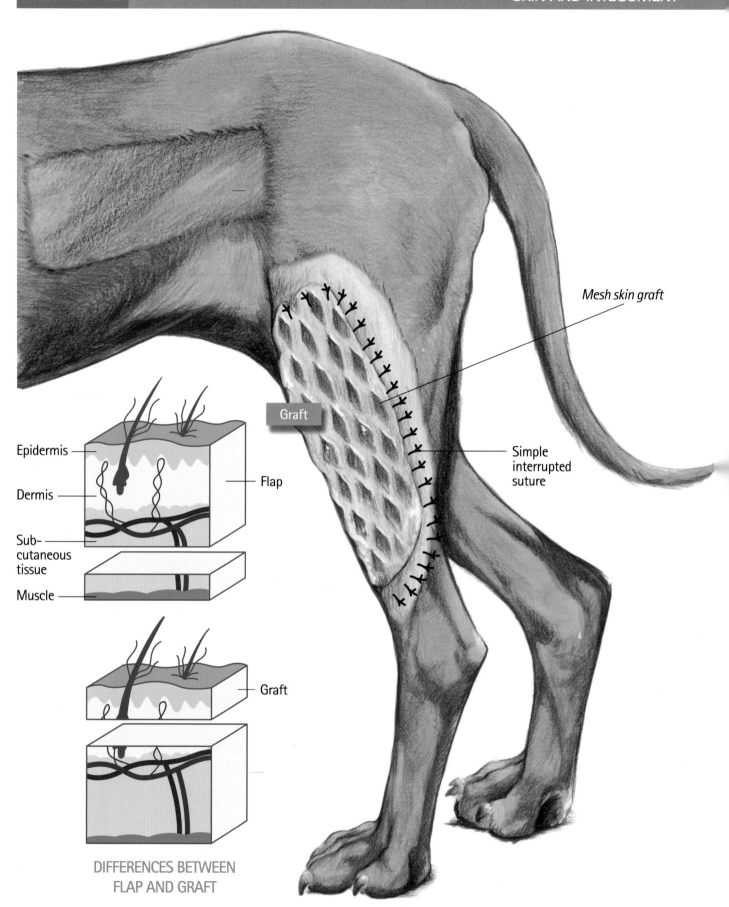

Mesh skin graft

Graft

Simple
interrupted
suture

Epidermis

Dermis

Sub-
cutaneous
tissue

Muscle

Flap

Graft

DIFFERENCES BETWEEN
FLAP AND GRAFT

Entropion

Illustration 2.1   EYE AND EYELIDS

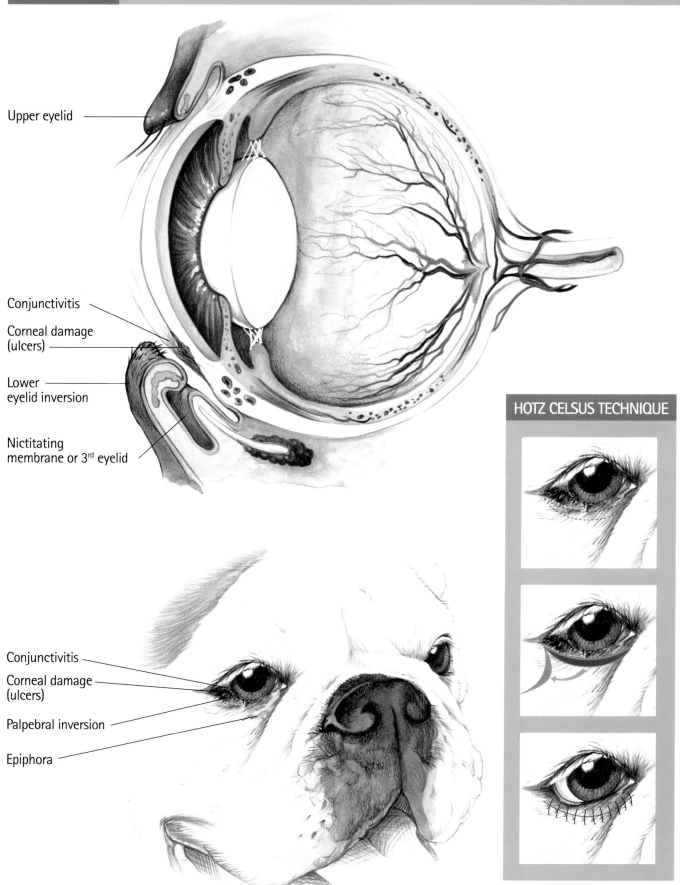

Upper eyelid

Conjunctivitis

Corneal damage (ulcers)

Lower eyelid inversion

Nictitating membrane or 3rd eyelid

Conjunctivitis

Corneal damage (ulcers)

Palpebral inversion

Epiphora

HOTZ CELSUS TECHNIQUE

Ectropion

Illustration 2.2

EYE AND EYELIDS

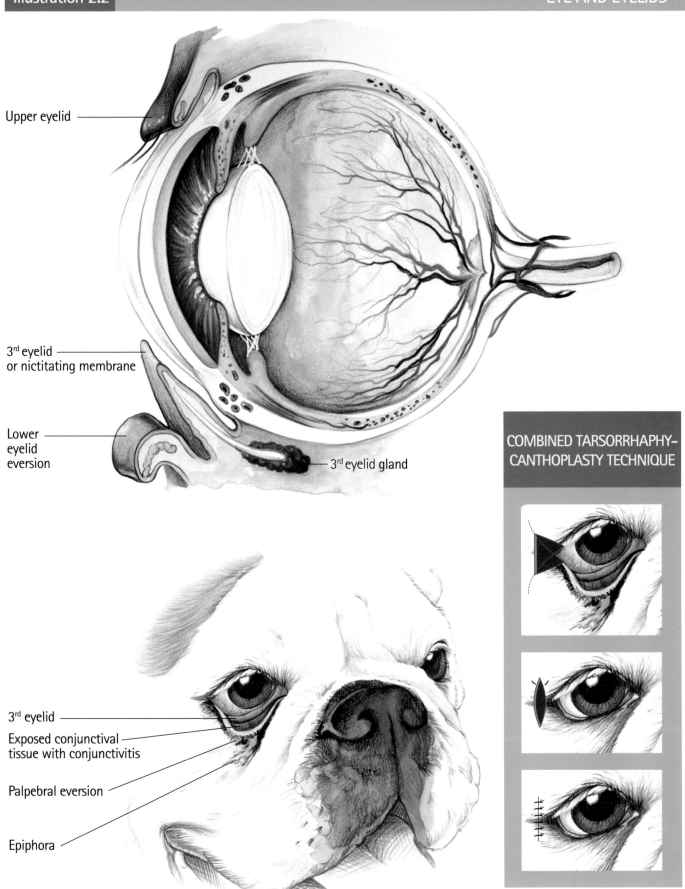

Upper eyelid

3rd eyelid
or nictitating membrane

Lower
eyelid
eversion

3rd eyelid gland

3rd eyelid

Exposed conjunctival
tissue with conjunctivitis

Palpebral eversion

Epiphora

COMBINED TARSORRHAPHY–CANTHOPLASTY TECHNIQUE

Prolapsed 3rd eyelid gland

Illustration 2.3   EYE AND EYELIDS

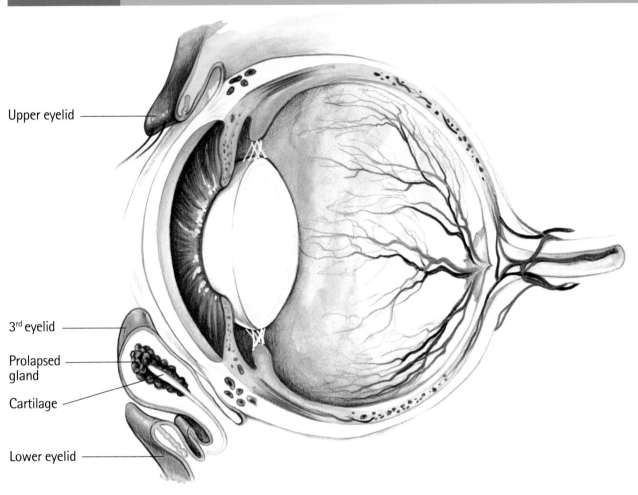

Upper eyelid

3rd eyelid

Prolapsed gland

Cartilage

Lower eyelid

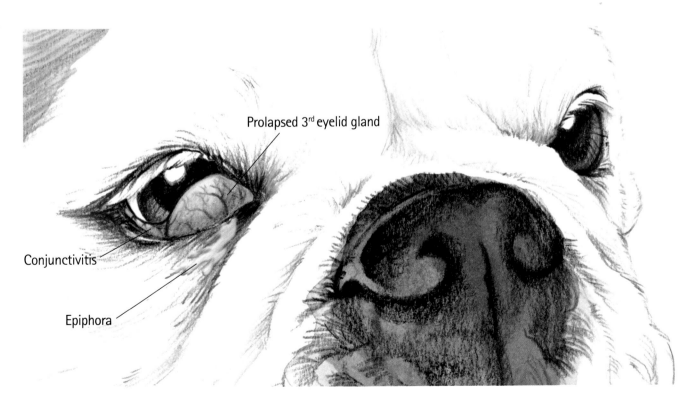

Prolapsed 3rd eyelid gland

Conjunctivitis

Epiphora

Eversion of the 3rd eyelid

Illustration 2.4   EYE AND EYELIDS

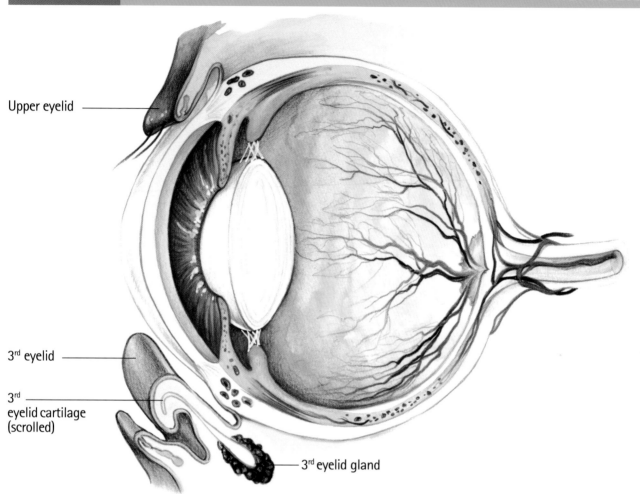

Upper eyelid

3rd eyelid

3rd eyelid cartilage (scrolled)

3rd eyelid gland

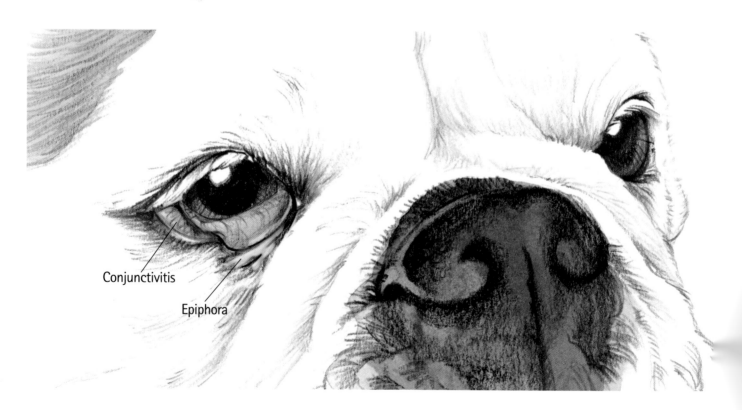

Conjunctivitis

Epiphora

Cataracts

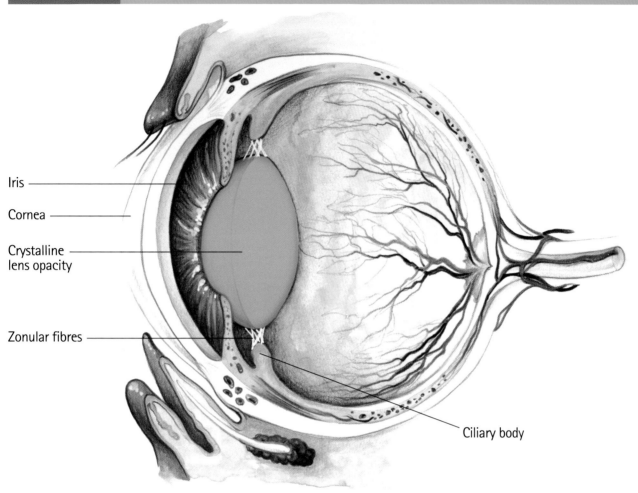

Iris

Cornea

Crystalline
lens opacity

Zonular fibres

Ciliary body

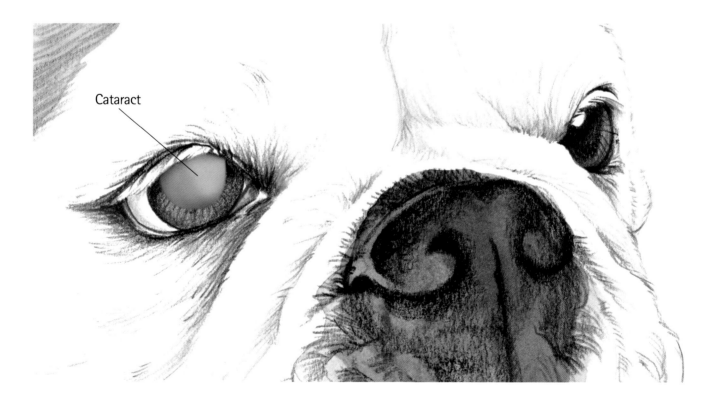

Cataract

Corneal ulcer

Illustration 2.6   EYE AND EYELIDS

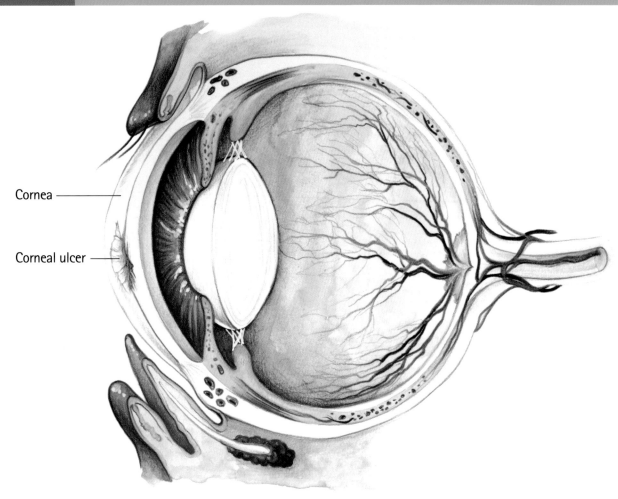

Cornea

Corneal ulcer

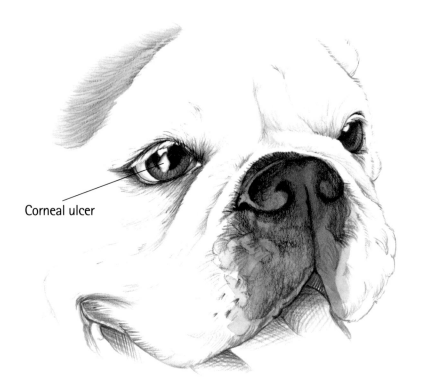

Corneal ulcer

NORMAL ULCER

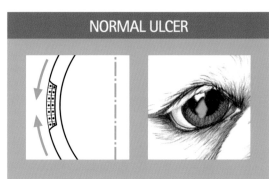

INDOLENT ULCER

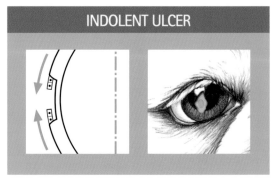

Ear canal ablation

Illustration 3.1

Inflammation

Chronic purulent otitis

Suppuration

Auricular cartilage

Suppuration

Epithelial inflammation of the auricular canal

Tympanic bulla osteotomy

Illustration 3.2   EAR AND PINNA

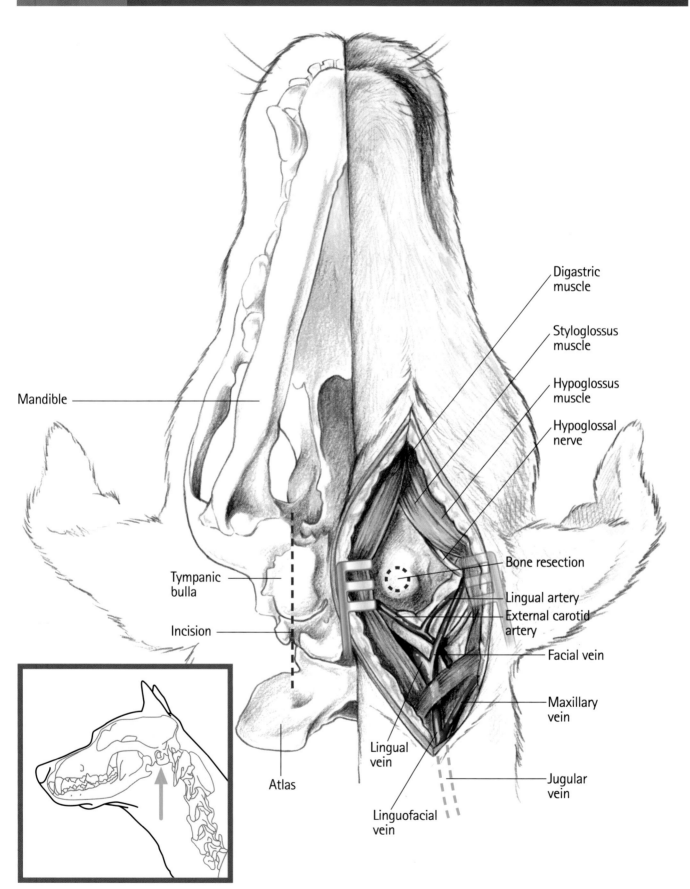

Digastric
muscle

Styloglossus
muscle

Hypoglossus
muscle

Hypoglossal
nerve

Mandible

Bone resection

Tympanic
bulla

Lingual artery

External carotid
artery

Incision

Facial vein

Maxillary
vein

Lingual
vein

Jugular
vein

Atlas

Linguofacial
vein

Aural haematoma

Illustration 3.3

Pinna

Anatomy of the abdominal cavity (dog)

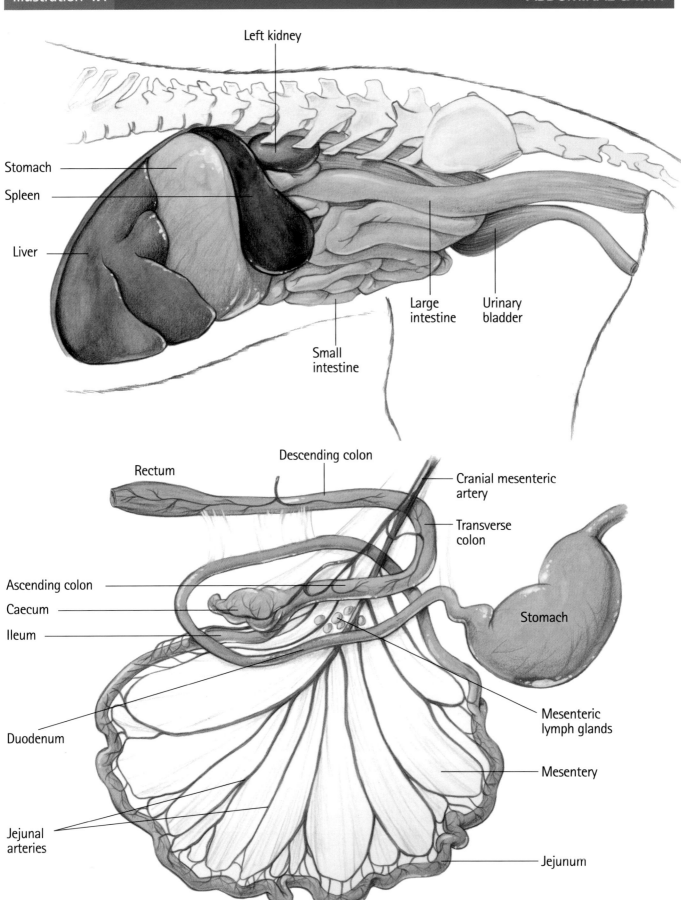

Left kidney

Stomach

Spleen

Liver

Large intestine

Urinary bladder

Small intestine

Descending colon

Rectum

Cranial mesenteric artery

Transverse colon

Ascending colon

Caecum

Ileum

Stomach

Duodenum

Mesenteric lymph glands

Mesentery

Jejunal arteries

Jejunum

Anatomy of the abdominal cavity (cat)

Illustration 4.2   ABDOMINAL CAVITY

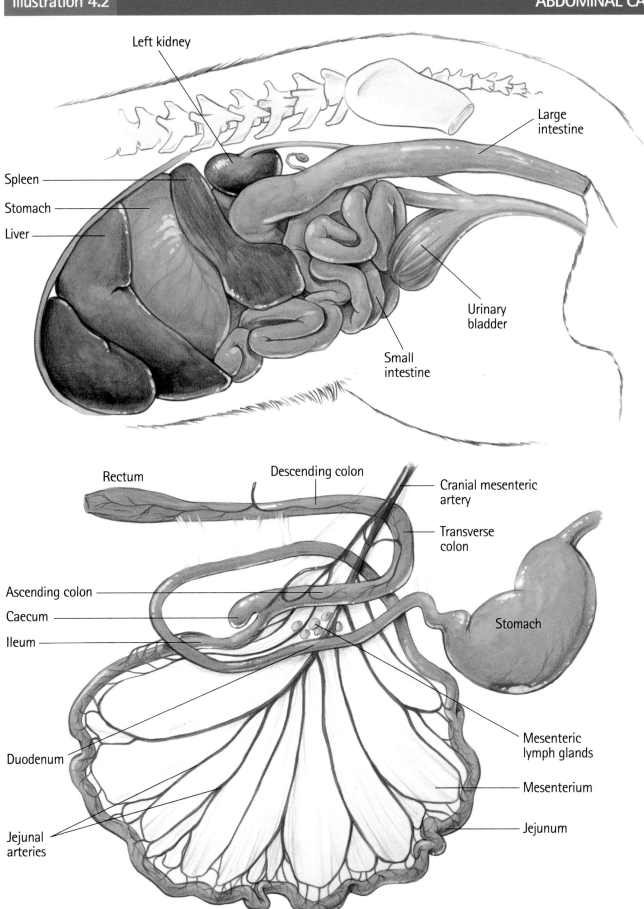

Left kidney

Large intestine

Spleen

Stomach

Liver

Urinary bladder

Small intestine

Rectum

Descending colon

Cranial mesenteric artery

Transverse colon

Ascending colon

Caecum

Ileum

Stomach

Mesenteric lymph glands

Mesenterium

Duodenum

Jejunum

Jejunal arteries

Umbilical hernia

Illustration 4.3   ABDOMINAL CAVITY

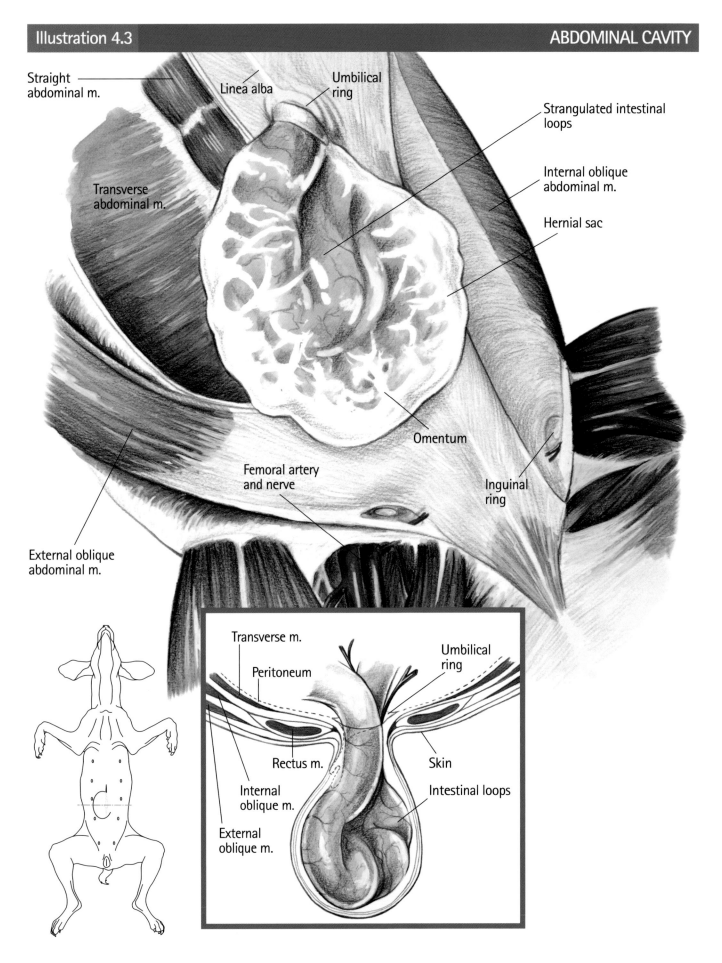

Straight abdominal m.

Linea alba

Umbilical ring

Strangulated intestinal loops

Internal oblique abdominal m.

Hernial sac

Transverse abdominal m.

Omentum

Femoral artery and nerve

Inguinal ring

External oblique abdominal m.

Transverse m.

Peritoneum

Umbilical ring

Rectus m.

Skin

Internal oblique m.

Intestinal loops

External oblique m.

Inguinal hernia

Illustration 4.4   ABDOMINAL CAVITY

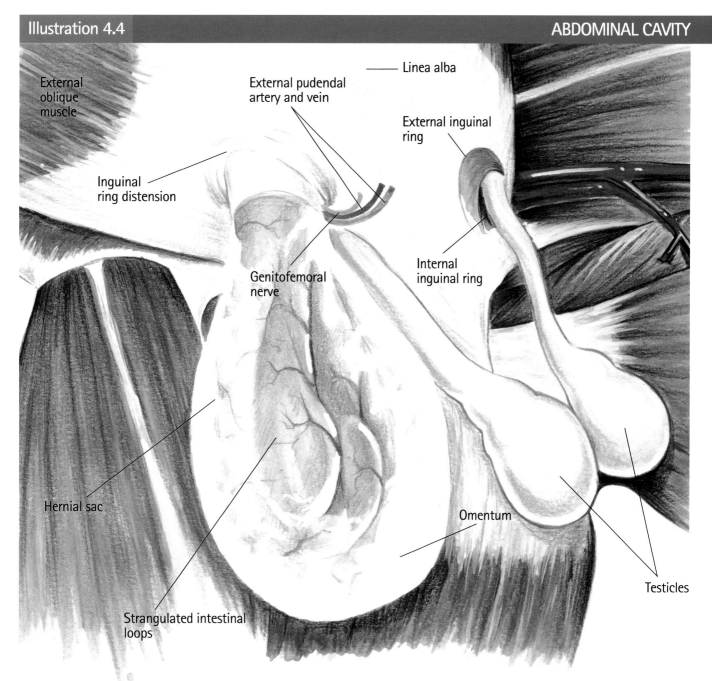

External oblique muscle

Inguinal ring distension

External pudendal artery and vein

Linea alba

External inguinal ring

Internal inguinal ring

Genitofemoral nerve

Hernial sac

Strangulated intestinal loops

Omentum

Testicles

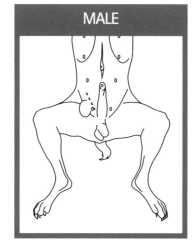

MALE

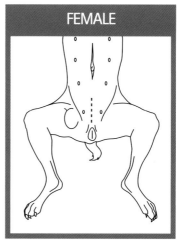

FEMALE

Normal canine teeth

Illustration 5.1   DIGESTIVE SYSTEM

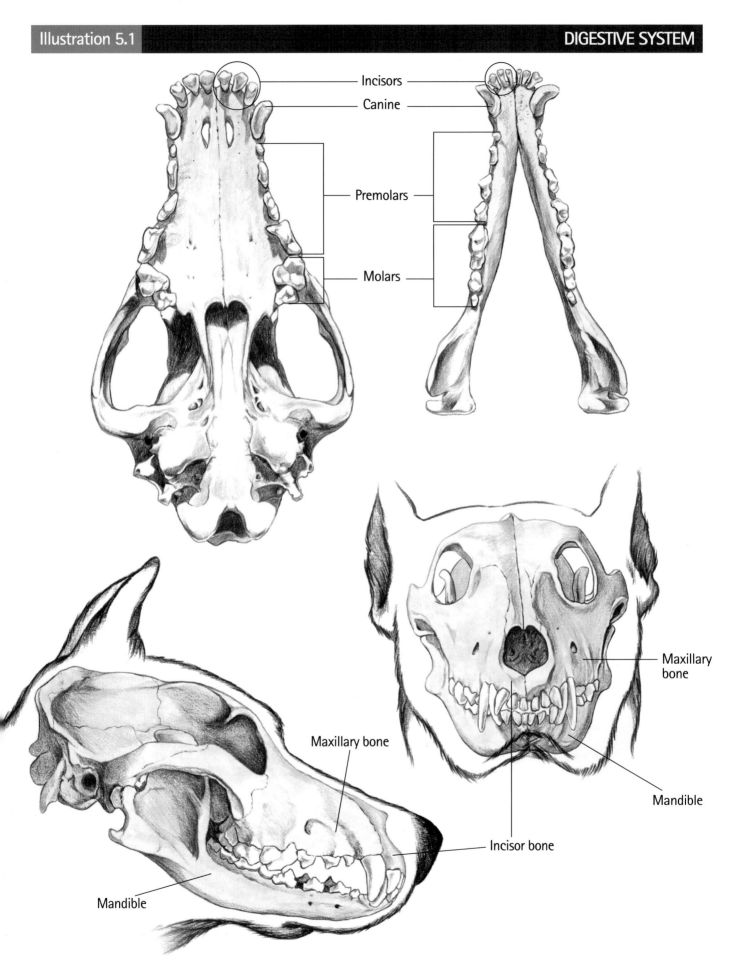

Incisors

Canine

Premolars

Molars

Maxillary bone

Maxillary bone

Mandible

Incisor bone

Mandible

Normal feline teeth

Illustration 5.2   DIGESTIVE SYSTEM

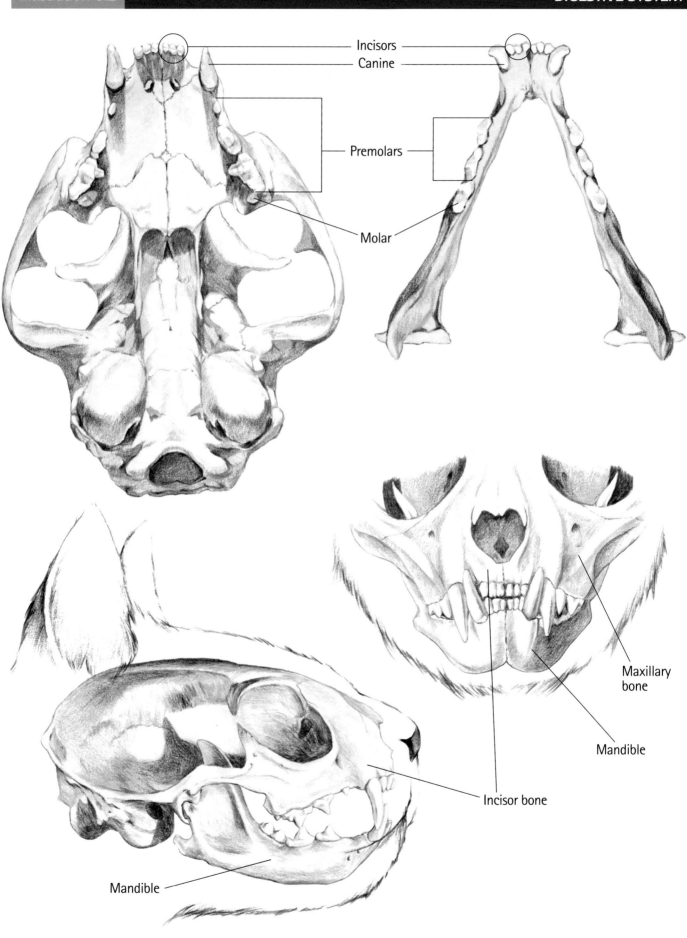

Incisors

Canine

Premolars

Molar

Maxillary bone

Mandible

Incisor bone

Mandible

Tartar and periodontal disease

Illustration 5.3

DIGESTIVE SYSTEM

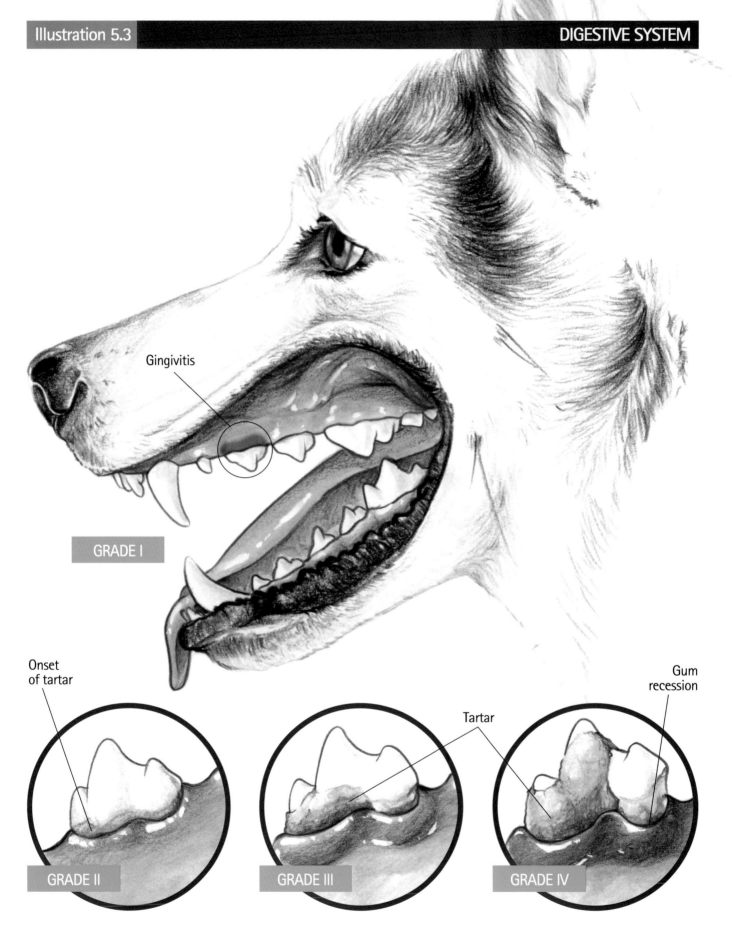

Gingivitis

GRADE I

Onset
of tartar

Tartar

Gum
recession

GRADE II

GRADE III

GRADE IV

Malar abscess

Illustration 5.4

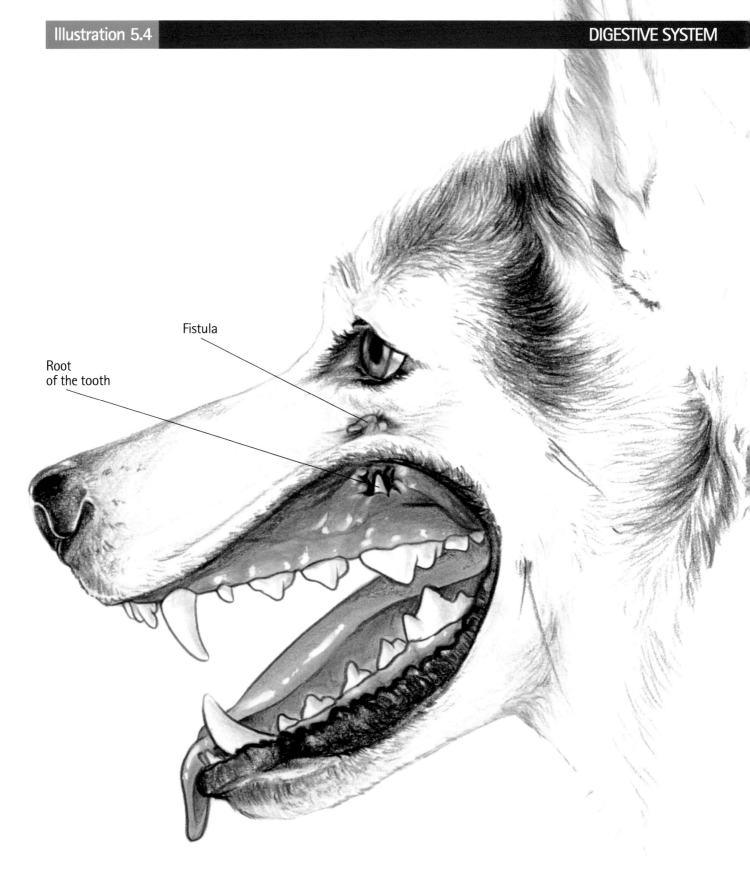

Fistula

Root
of the tooth

Oronasal fistula and palatine groove

Illustration 5.5 | DIGESTIVE SYSTEM

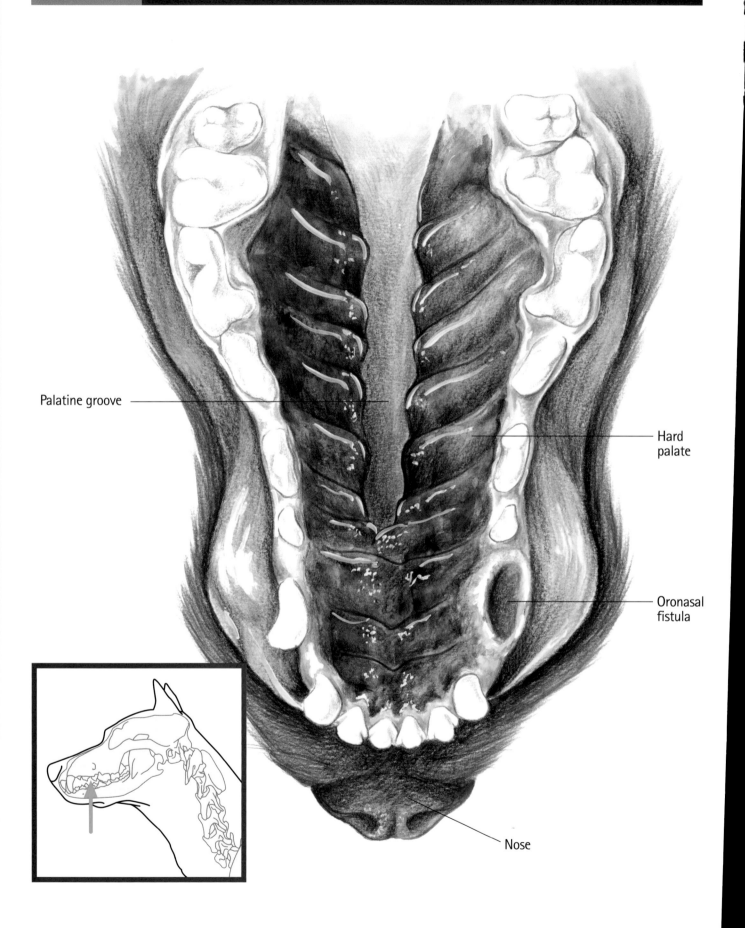

Palatine groove

Hard palate

Oronasal fistula

Nose

Oesophageal foreign body

Illustration 5.6   DIGESTIVE SYSTEM

Trachea

Foreign body
(ball, toy)

Oesophagus

Proximal dilation

Oesophagitis

Mucosal necrosis

Heart

Oesophageal stenosis

Illustration 5.7

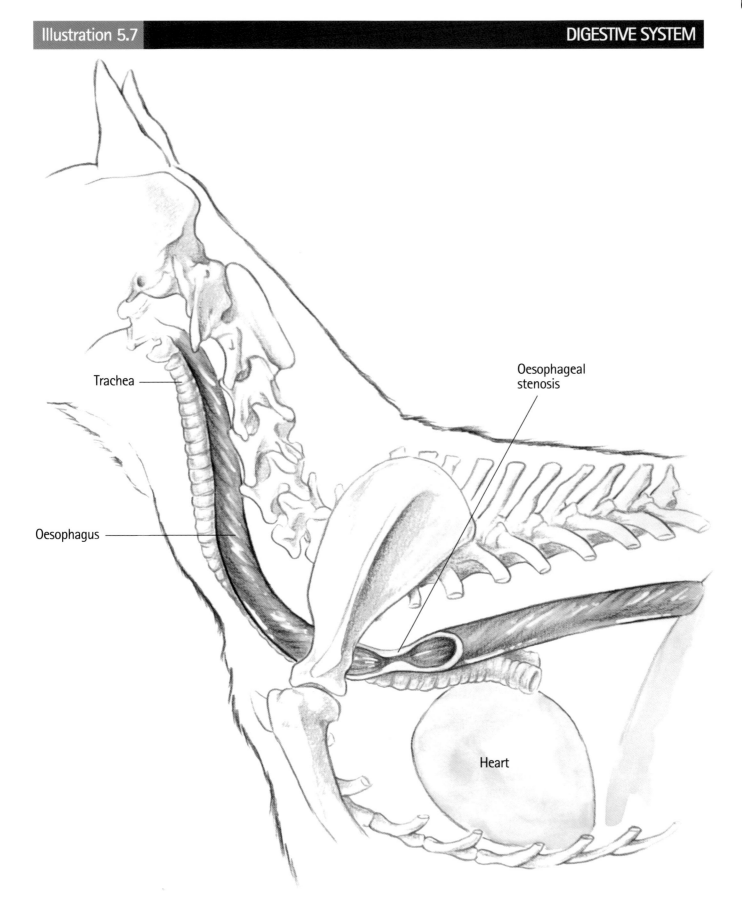

Trachea

Oesophagus

Oesophageal
stenosis

Heart

Oesophageal diverticulum

Illustration 5.8

Trachea

Oesophageal diverticulum

Oesophagus

Heart

Tracheal bifurcation

Hiatus hernia

Illustration 5.9

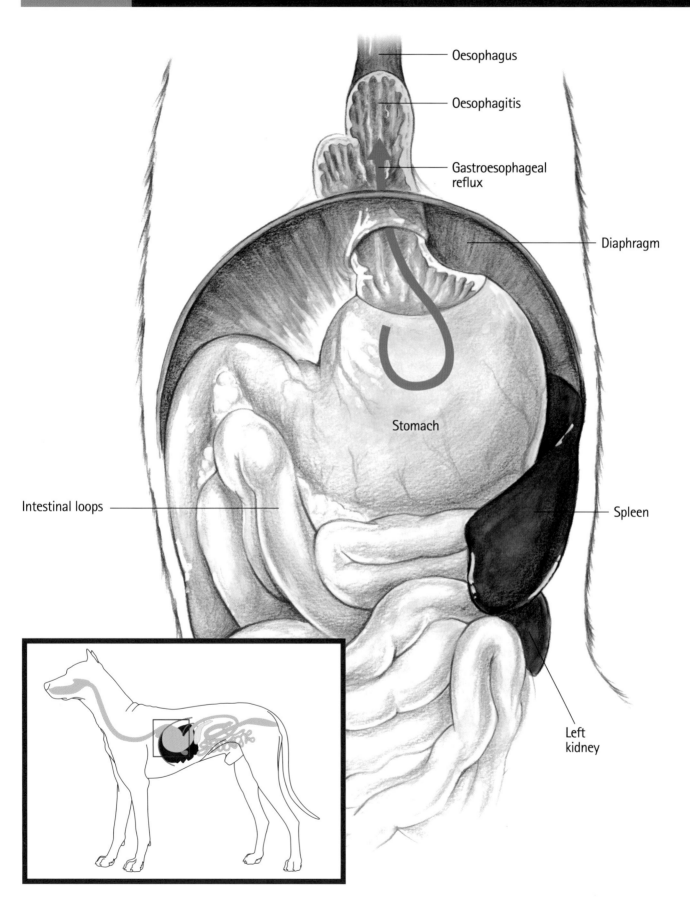

Oesophagus

Oesophagitis

Gastroesophageal reflux

Diaphragm

Stomach

Intestinal loops

Spleen

Left kidney

Persistent right aortic arch (PRRA)

Illustration 5.10 DIGESTIVE SYSTEM

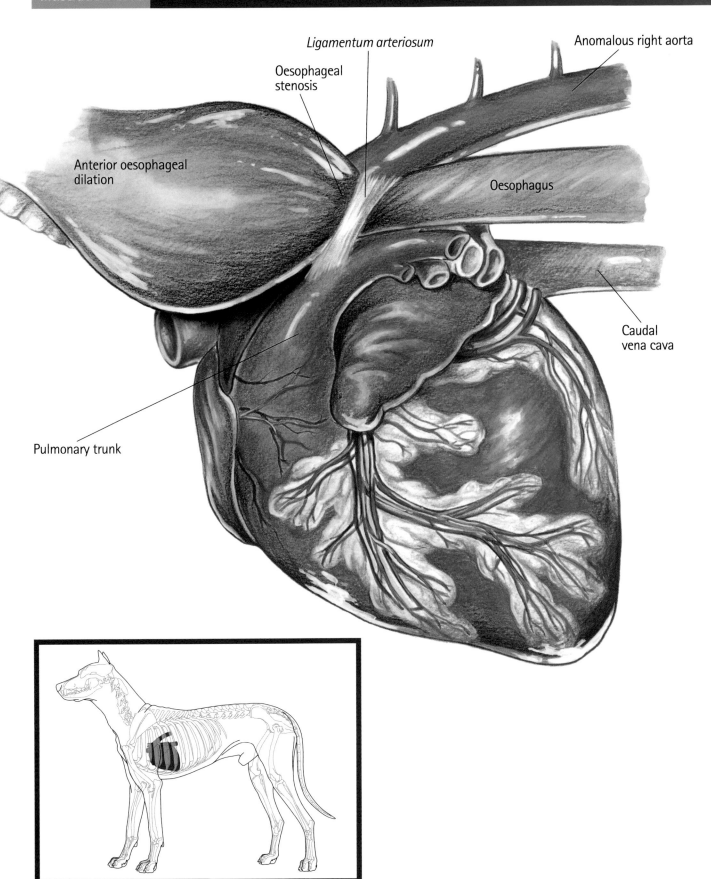

Ligamentum arteriosum

Oesophageal stenosis

Anomalous right aorta

Anterior oesophageal dilation

Oesophagus

Caudal vena cava

Pulmonary trunk

Gastric foreign body Gastrotomy

Illustration 5.11   DIGESTIVE SYSTEM

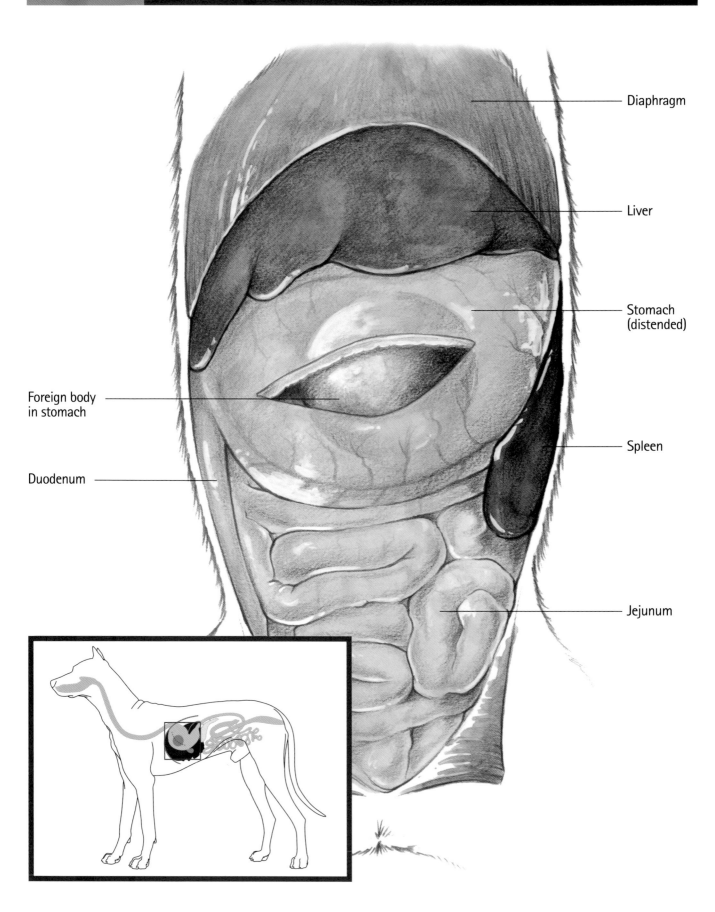

Diaphragm

Liver

Stomach (distended)

Foreign body in stomach

Spleen

Duodenum

Jejunum

Gastric dilatation–volvulus Gastropexy

Illustration 5.12   DIGESTIVE SYSTEM

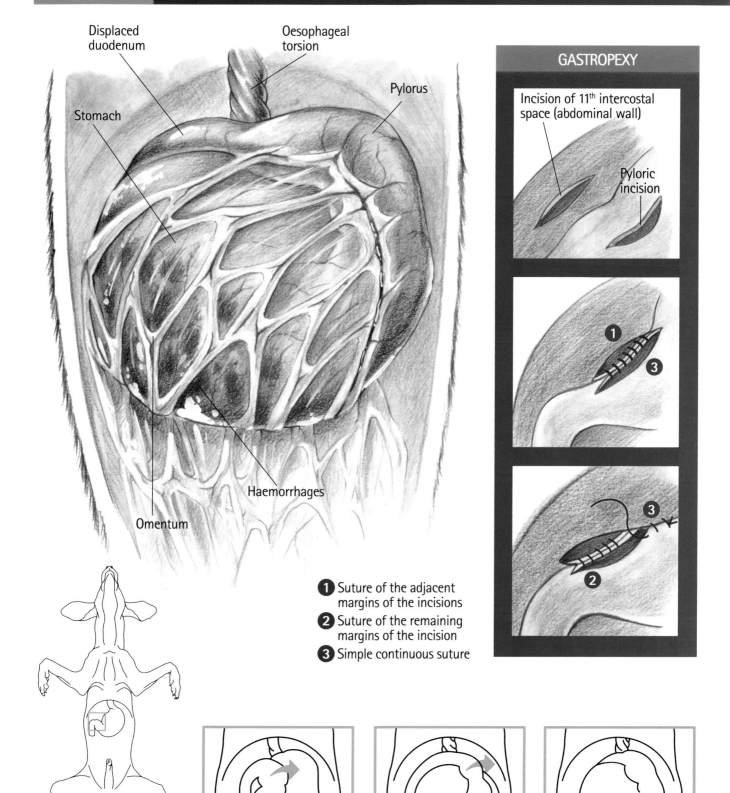

Displaced duodenum

Oesophageal torsion

Pylorus

Stomach

Haemorrhages

Omentum

Gastropexy zone

GASTROPEXY

Incision of 11th intercostal space (abdominal wall)

Pyloric incision

1

3

3

2

1 Suture of the adjacent margins of the incisions

2 Suture of the remaining margins of the incision

3 Simple continuous suture

1

2

3

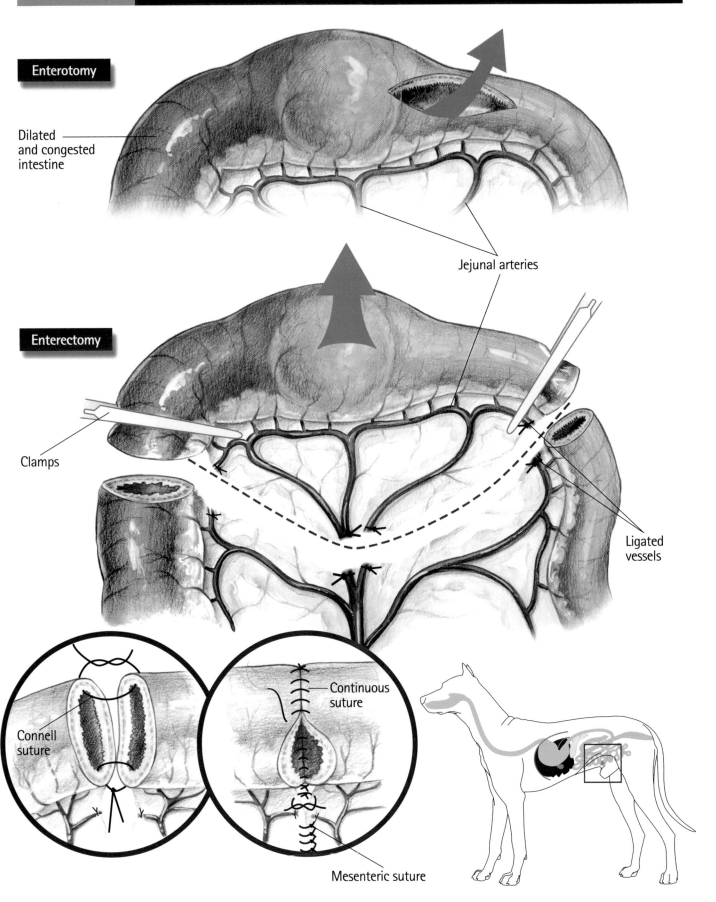

Enterotomy

Dilated and congested intestine

Jejunal arteries

Enterectomy

Clamps

Ligated vessels

Connell suture

Continuous suture

Mesenteric suture

Intestinal intussusception

Illustration 5.14

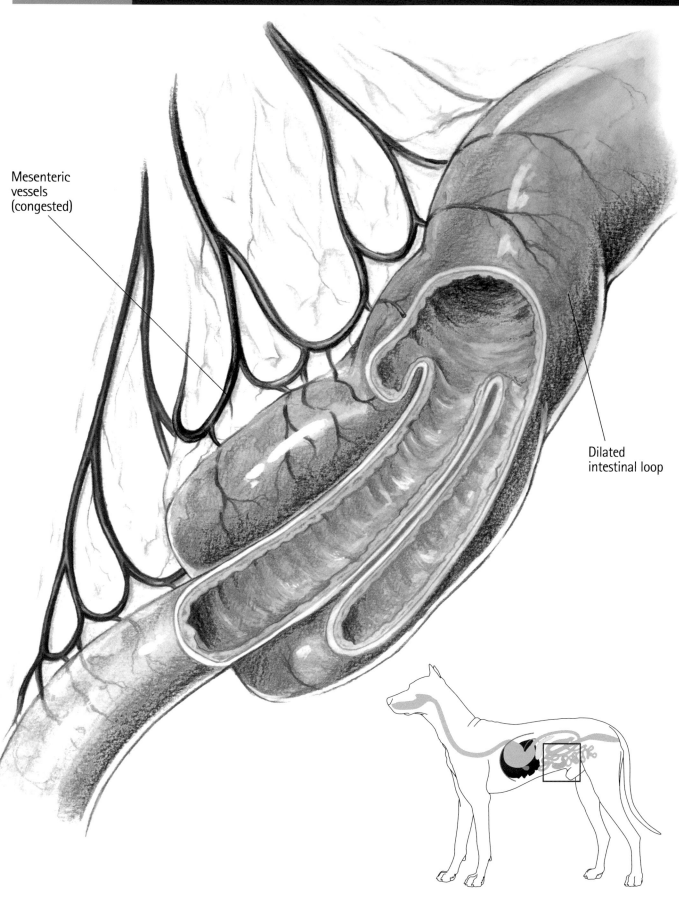

Mesenteric
vessels
(congested)

Dilated
intestinal loop

Intestinal volvulus/Torsion

Illustration 5.15

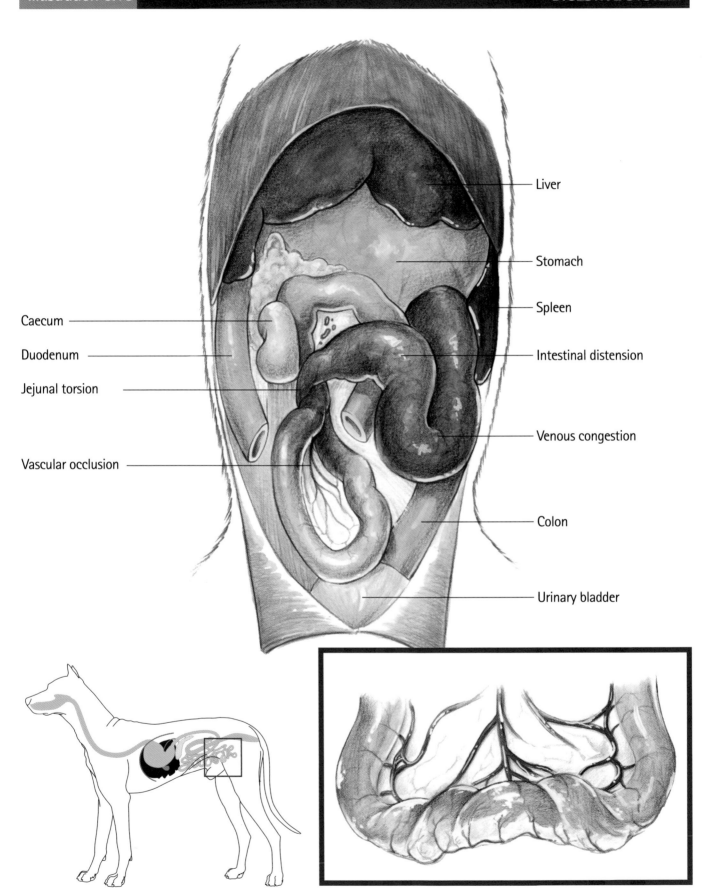

Liver

Stomach

Spleen

Intestinal distension

Venous congestion

Colon

Urinary bladder

Caecum

Duodenum

Jejunal torsion

Vascular occlusion

Megacolon

Illustration 5.16

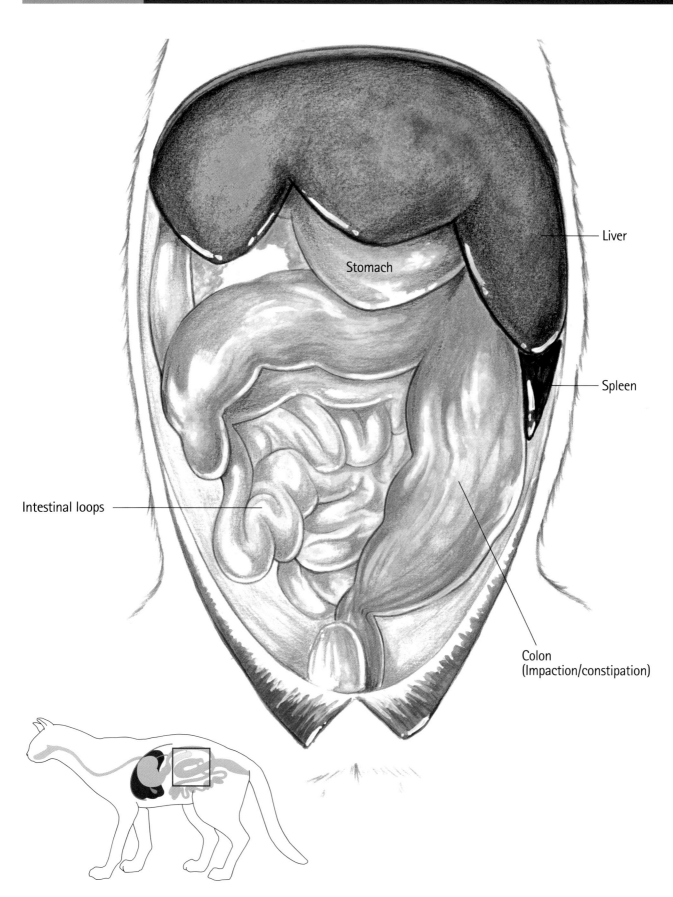

Liver

Stomach

Spleen

Intestinal loops

Colon
(Impaction/constipation)

Infection /Impaction of the anal sacs

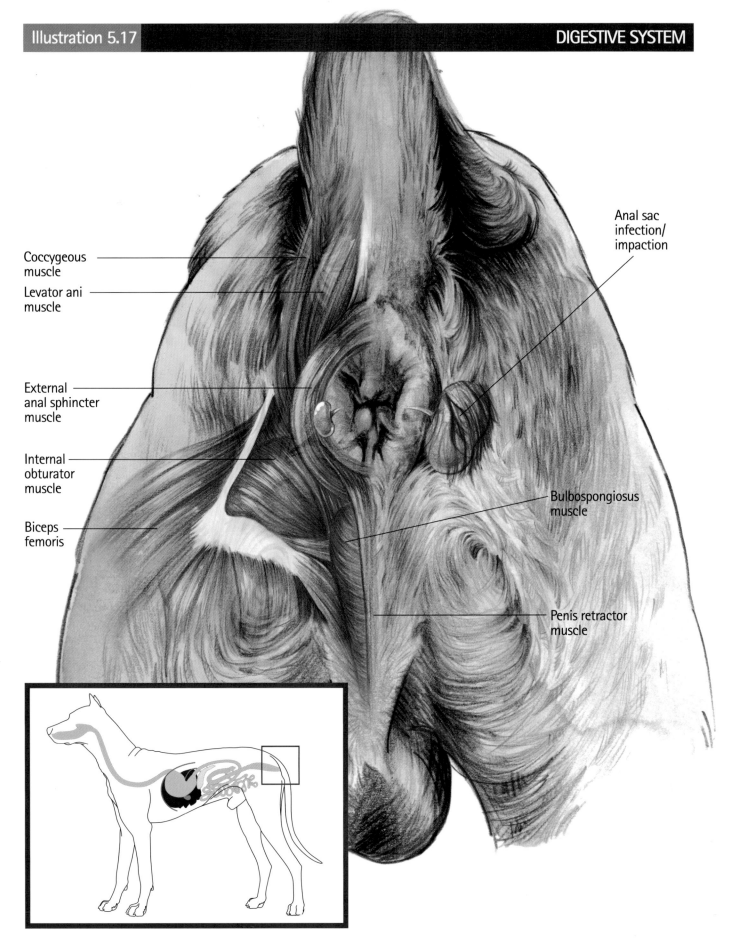

Coccygeous muscle

Levator ani muscle

External anal sphincter muscle

Internal obturator muscle

Biceps femoris

Anal sac infection/ impaction

Bulbospongiosus muscle

Penis retractor muscle

Perineal hernia

Illustration 5.18   DIGESTIVE SYSTEM

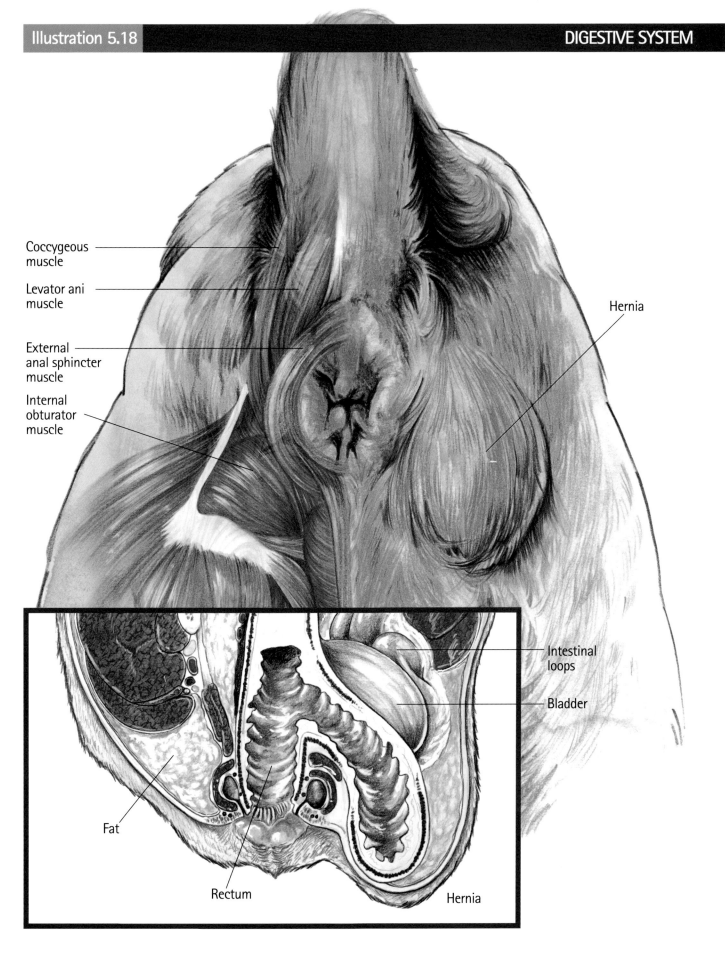

Coccygeous muscle

Levator ani muscle

External anal sphincter muscle

Internal obturator muscle

Hernia

Intestinal loops

Bladder

Fat

Rectum

Hernia

Perianal fistulas

Illustration 5.19

Perianal
fistulas

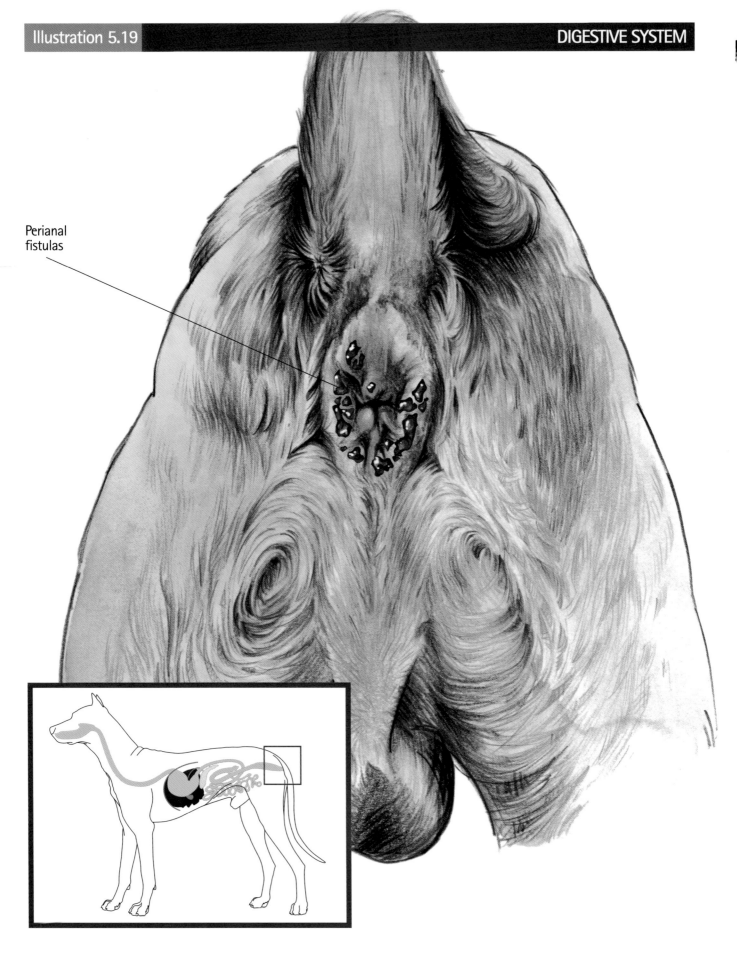

Rectal prolapse

Illustration 5.20

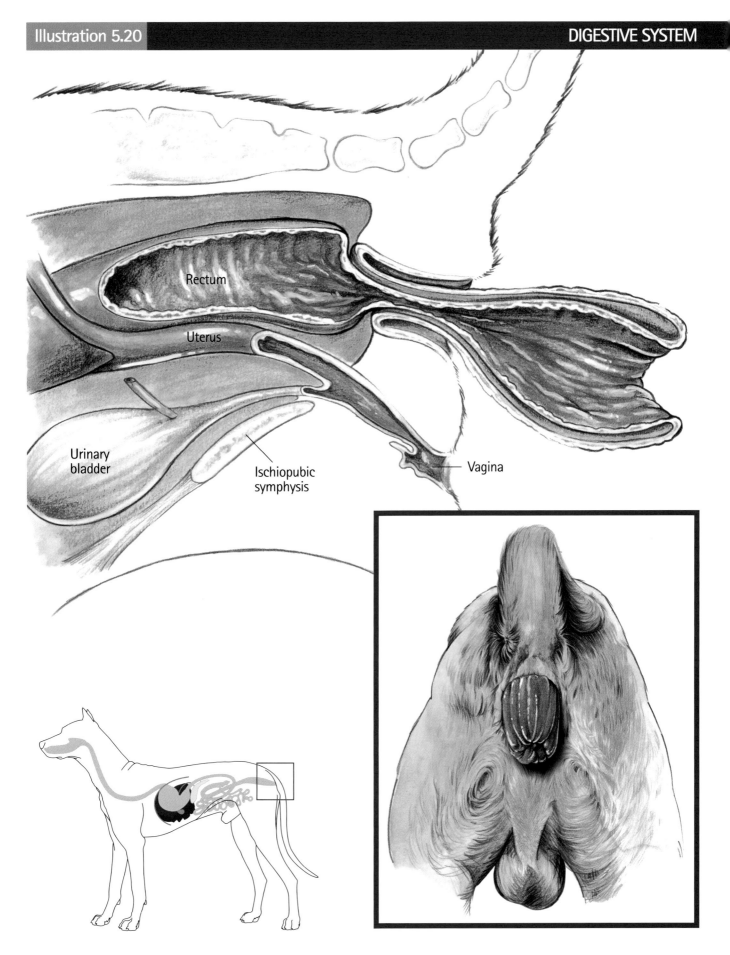

Rectum

Uterus

Urinary
bladder

Ischiopubic
symphysis

Vagina

Hepatic neoplasia Partial lobectomy

Illustration 5.21

Abdominal aorta

Caudal caval vein

Oesophagus

Neoplastic
areas

Liver

Suture

Portal vein

Gallbladder

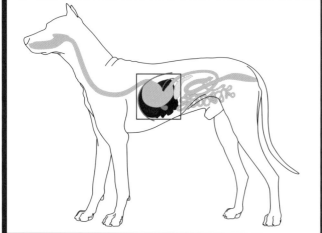

Cholelithiasis (Gallstones)

Illustration 5.22   DIGESTIVE SYSTEM

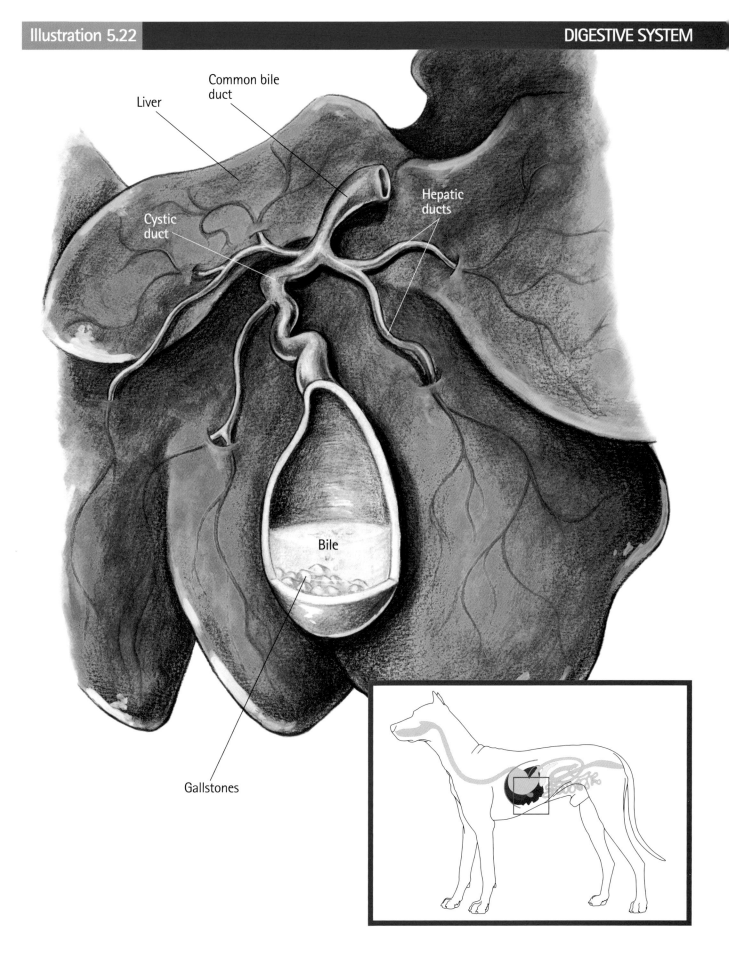

Liver

Common bile
duct

Cystic
duct

Hepatic
ducts

Bile

Gallstones

Adrenal neoplasia Adrenalectomy

Illustration 6.1

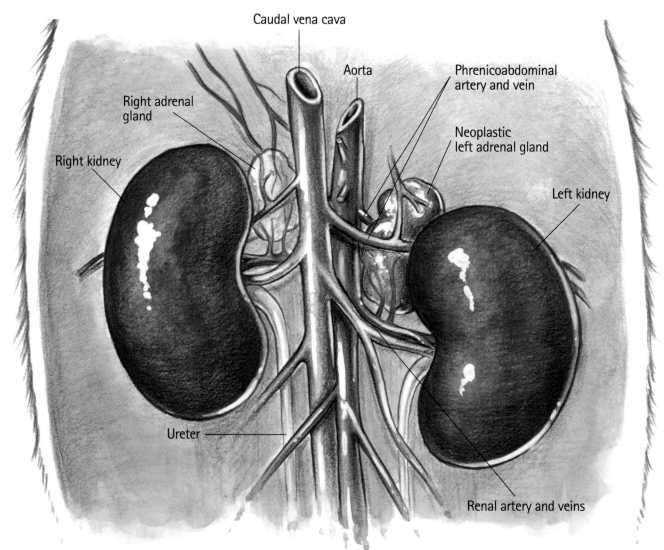

Caudal vena cava

Aorta

Phrenicoabdominal artery and vein

Right adrenal gland

Neoplastic left adrenal gland

Right kidney

Left kidney

Ureter

Renal artery and veins

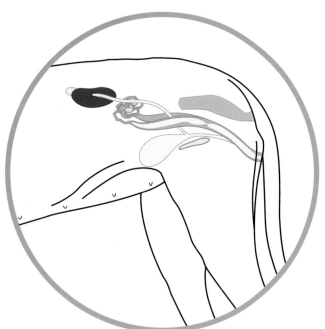

CUSHING'S SYNDROME

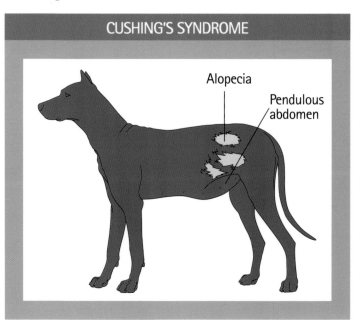

Alopecia

Pendulous abdomen

Hypophyseal neoplasia

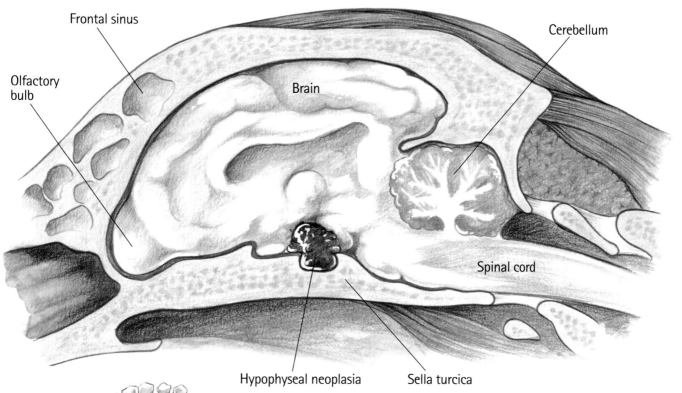

Frontal sinus

Cerebellum

Olfactory bulb

Brain

Spinal cord

Hypophyseal neoplasia

Sella turcica

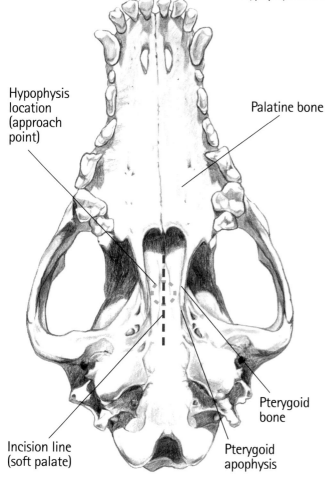

Hypophysis location (approach point)

Palatine bone

Pterygoid bone

Incision line (soft palate)

Pterygoid apophysis

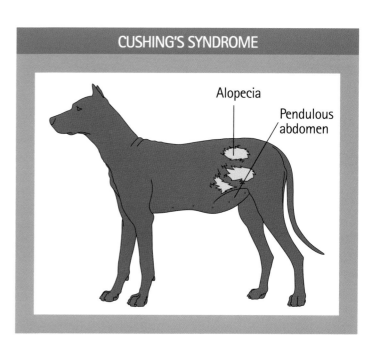

CUSHING'S SYNDROME

Alopecia

Pendulous abdomen

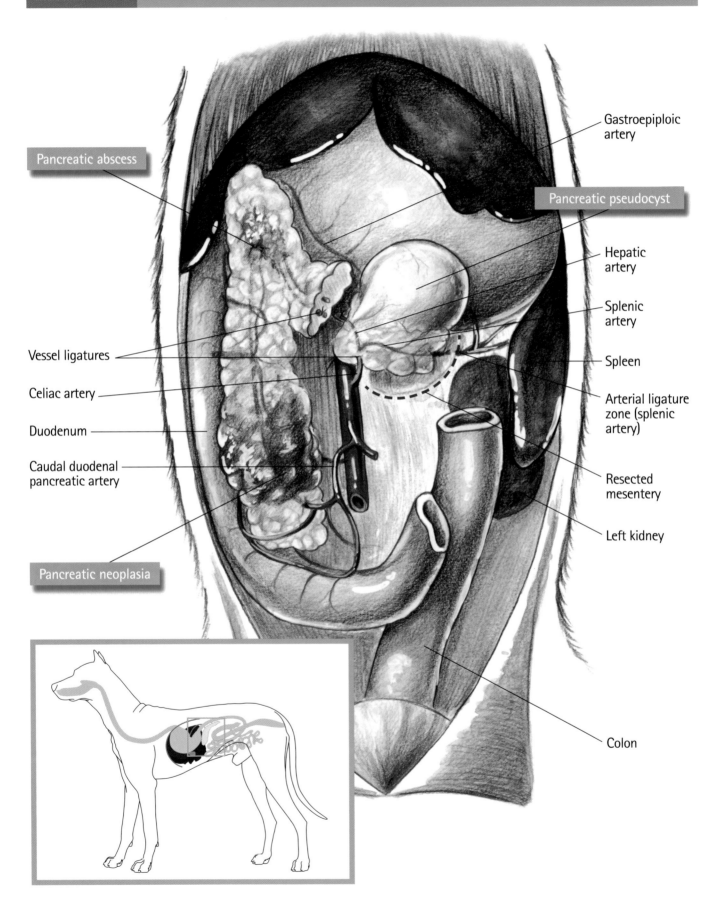

Pancreatic abscess

Gastroepiploic artery

Pancreatic pseudocyst

Hepatic artery

Splenic artery

Vessel ligatures

Spleen

Celiac artery

Arterial ligature zone (splenic artery)

Duodenum

Caudal duodenal pancreatic artery

Resected mesentery

Left kidney

Pancreatic neoplasia

Colon

Feline hyperthyroidism Thyroidectomy

Illustration 6.4　　　　　　　　ENDOCRINE AND HAEMOLYMPHATIC SYSTEM

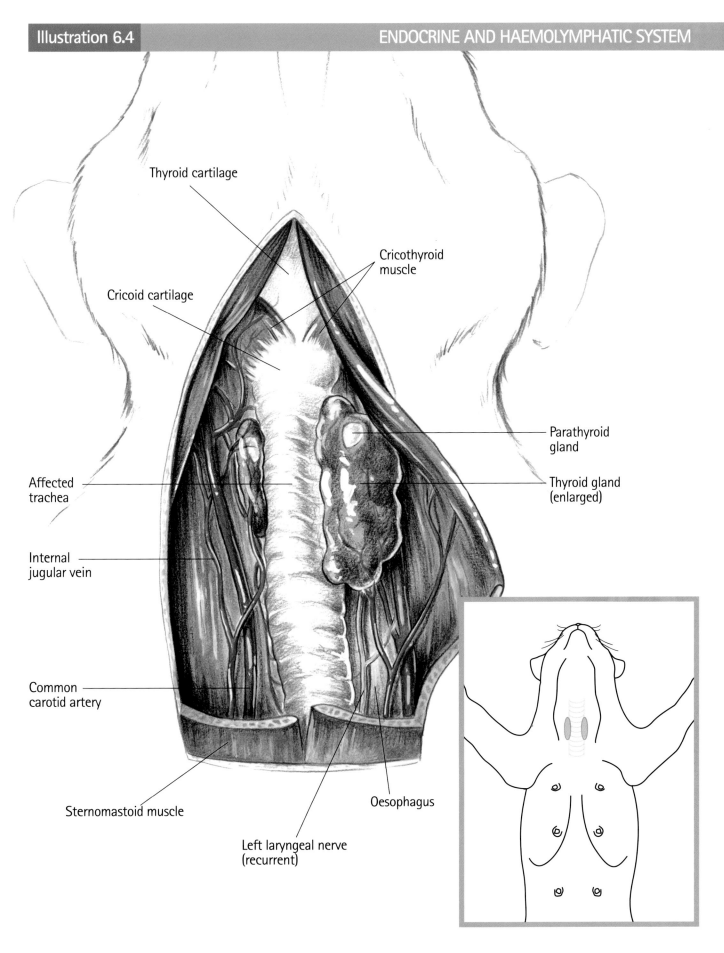

Thyroid cartilage

Cricothyroid muscle

Cricoid cartilage

Parathyroid gland

Thyroid gland (enlarged)

Affected trachea

Internal jugular vein

Common carotid artery

Sternomastoid muscle

Oesophagus

Left laryngeal nerve (recurrent)

Splenic torsion

Illustration 6.5   ENDOCRINE AND HAEMOLYMPHATIC SYSTEM

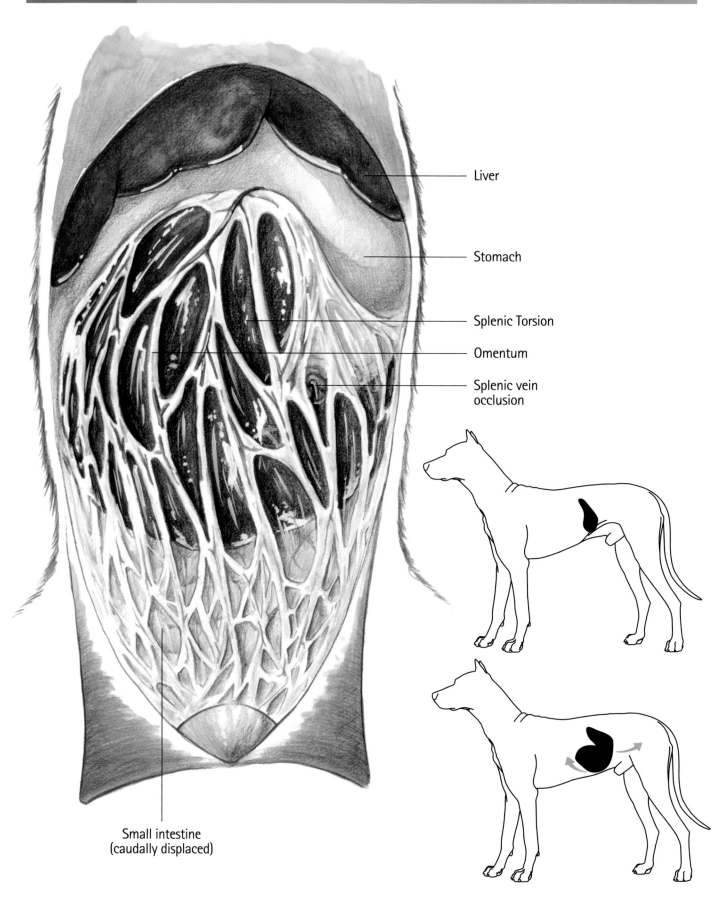

Liver

Stomach

Splenic Torsion

Omentum

Splenic vein
occlusion

Small intestine
(caudally displaced)

SPLENOMEGALY–TORSION

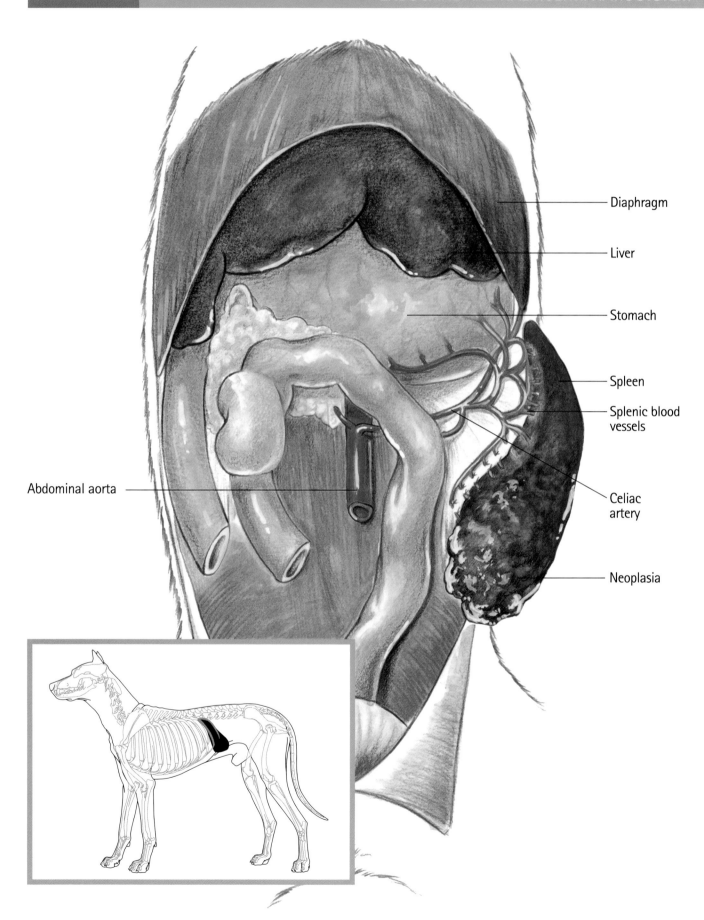

Diaphragm

Liver

Stomach

Spleen

Splenic blood vessels

Celiac artery

Neoplasia

Abdominal aorta

Ectopic ureter

Illustration 7.1   UROGENITAL SYSTEM

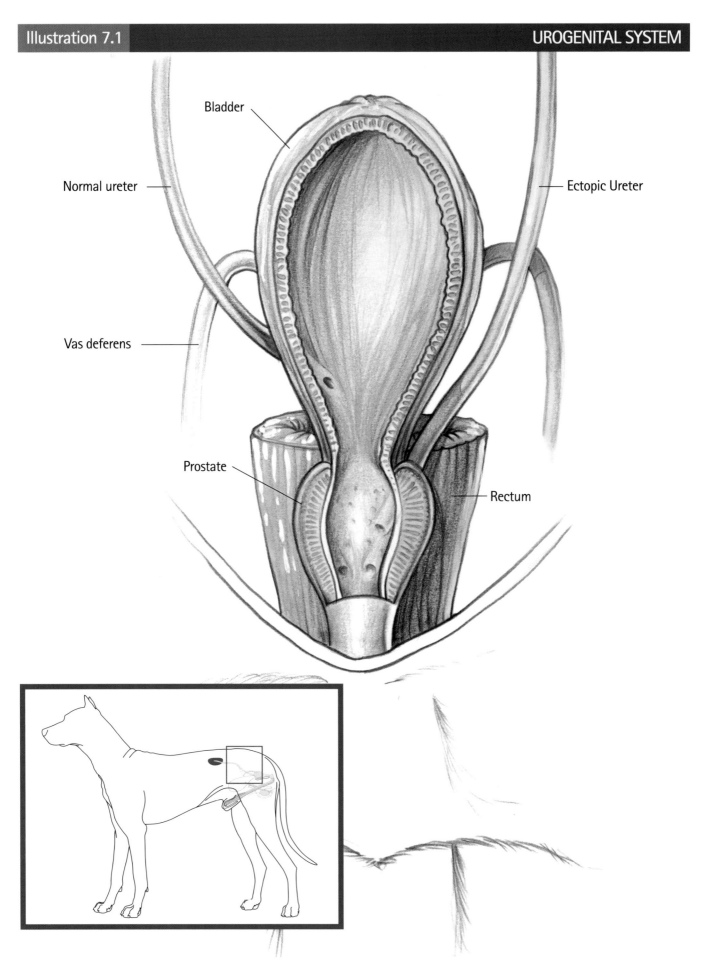

Bladder

Normal ureter

Ectopic Ureter

Vas deferens

Prostate

Rectum

Urolithiasis or kidney stones
(Kidney, ureter and bladder)

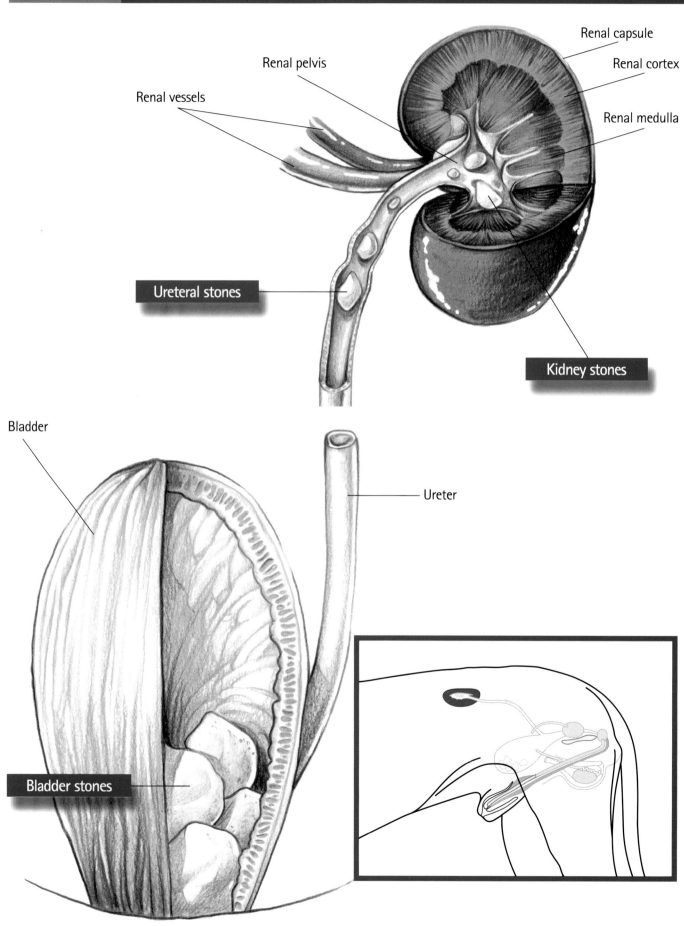

Renal pelvis

Renal vessels

Renal capsule

Renal cortex

Renal medulla

Ureteral stones

Kidney stones

Bladder

Ureter

Bladder stones

FLUTD (Feline Lower Urinary Tract Disease)

Illustration 7.3   UROGENITAL SYSTEM

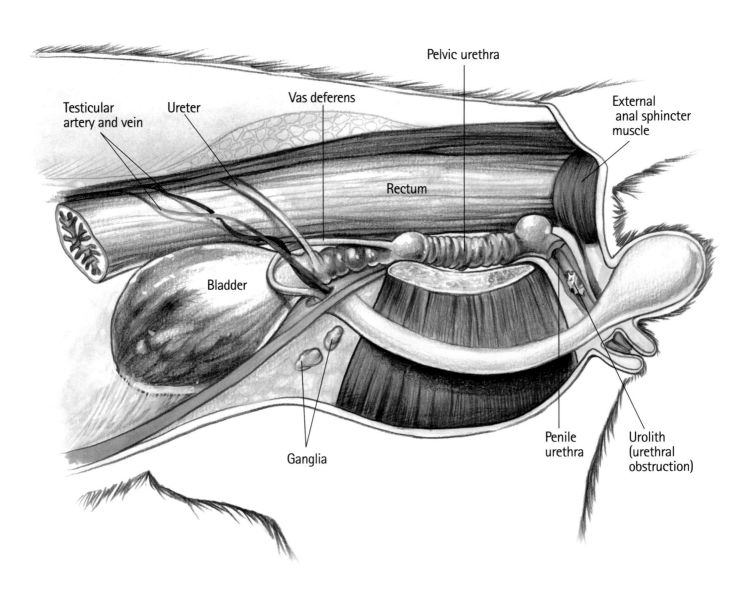

Pelvic urethra

Vas deferens

External anal sphincter muscle

Testicular artery and vein

Ureter

Rectum

Bladder

Ganglia

Penile urethra

Urolith (urethral obstruction)

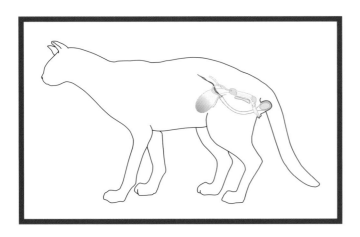

Ovariohysterectomy

Illustration 7.4

UROGENITAL SYSTEM

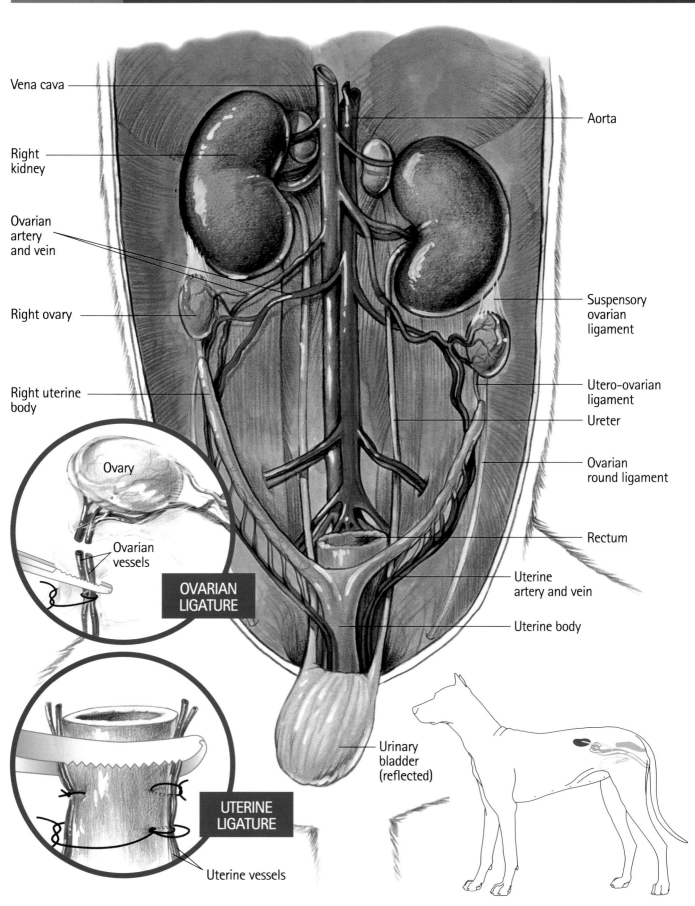

Vena cava

Aorta

Right kidney

Ovarian artery and vein

Right ovary

Suspensory ovarian ligament

Right uterine body

Utero-ovarian ligament

Ureter

Ovarian round ligament

Ovary

Ovarian vessels

OVARIAN LIGATURE

Rectum

Uterine artery and vein

Uterine body

UTERINE LIGATURE

Uterine vessels

Urinary bladder (reflected)

Canine/Feline orchidectomy

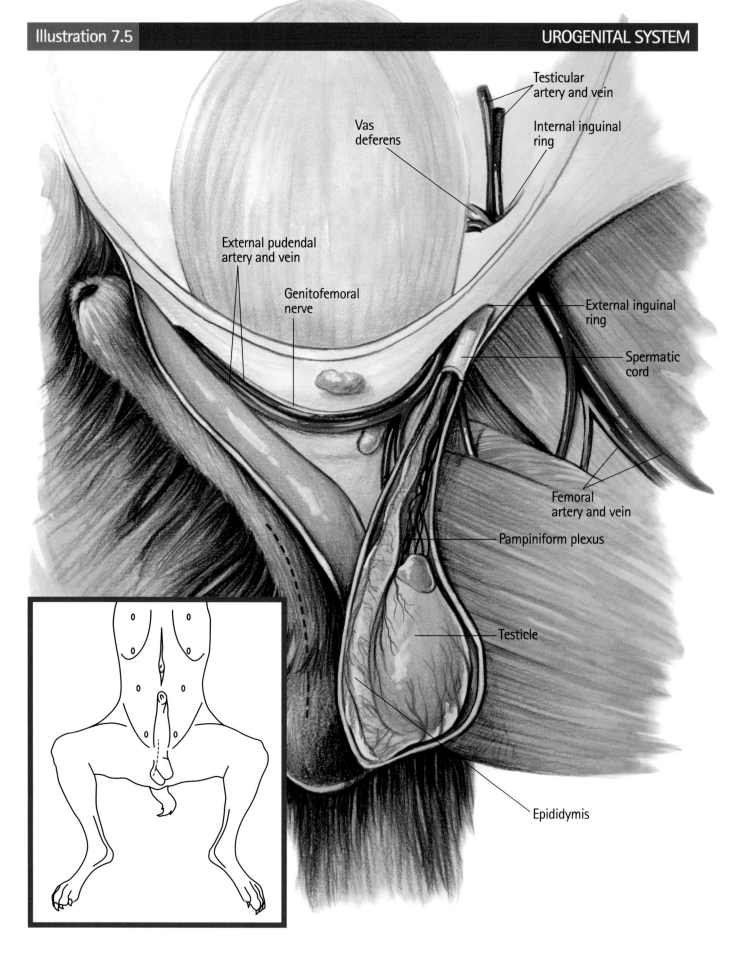

Testicular artery and vein

Vas deferens

Internal inguinal ring

External pudendal artery and vein

Genitofemoral nerve

External inguinal ring

Spermatic cord

Femoral artery and vein

Pampiniform plexus

Testicle

Epididymis

Caesarean section

Illustration 7.6   UROGENITAL SYSTEM

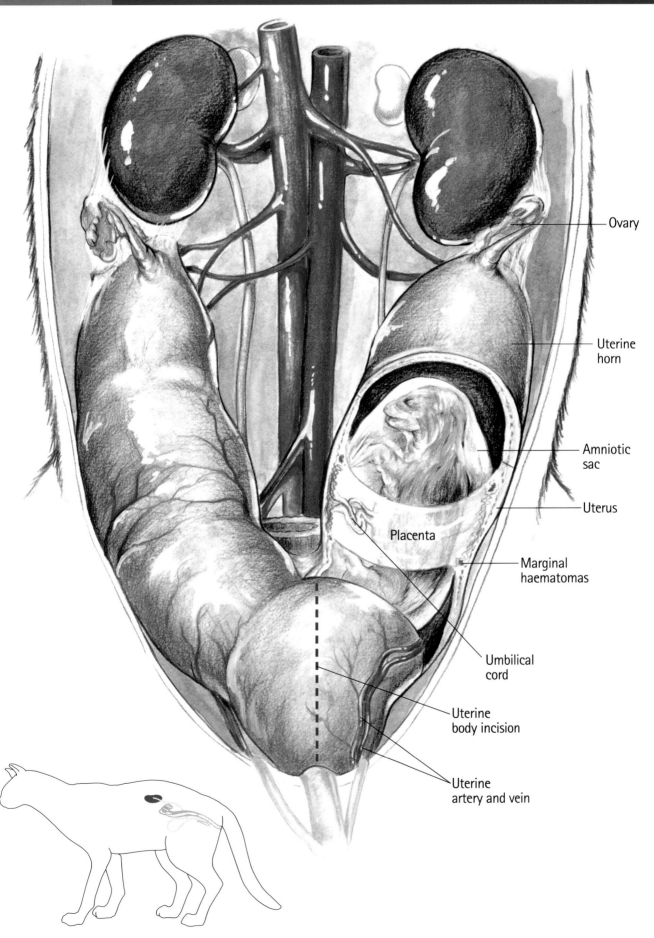

Ovary

Uterine horn

Amniotic sac

Uterus

Placenta

Marginal haematomas

Umbilical cord

Uterine body incision

Uterine artery and vein

Prostatic neoplasia/abscess/hyperplasia
Prostatectomy

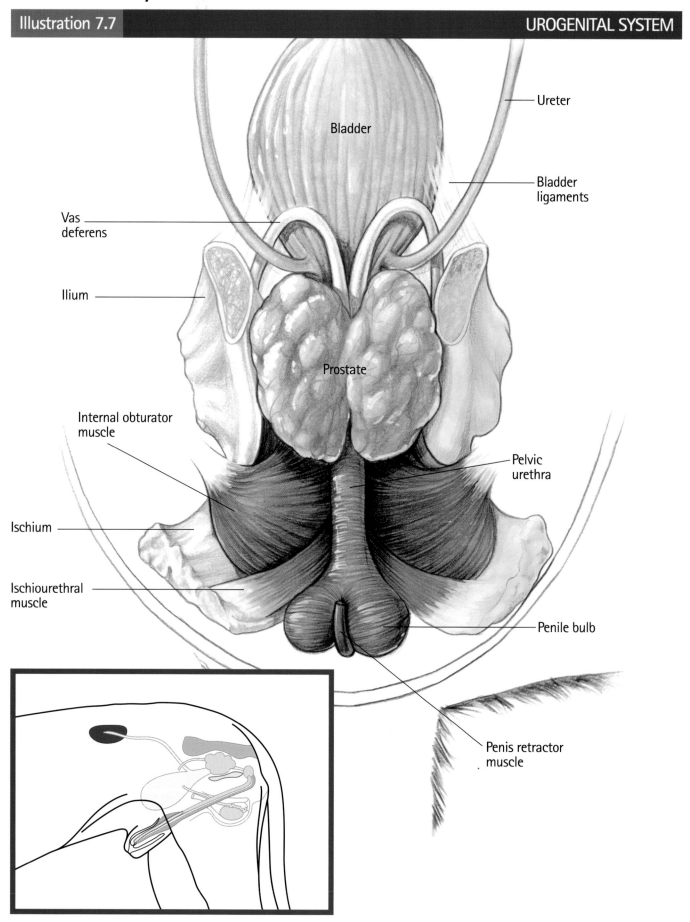

Ureter

Bladder

Bladder ligaments

Vas deferens

Ilium

Prostate

Internal obturator muscle

Pelvic urethra

Ischium

Ischiourethral muscle

Penile bulb

Penis retractor muscle

Mammary gland neoplasia Mastectomy

Illustration 7.8

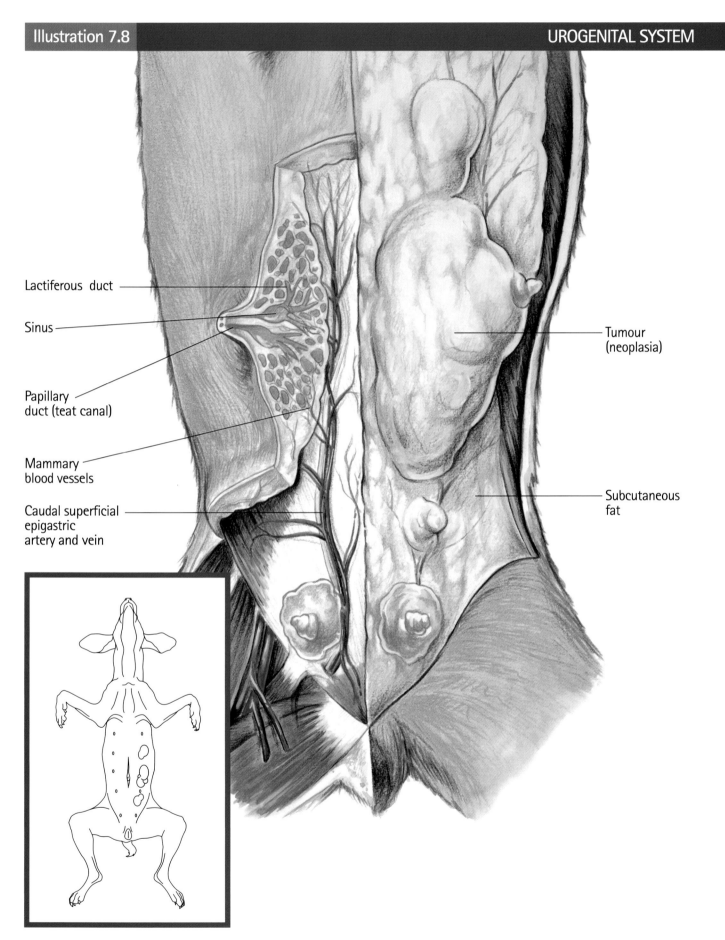

Lactiferous duct

Sinus

Papillary duct (teat canal)

Mammary blood vessels

Caudal superficial epigastric artery and vein

Tumour (neoplasia)

Subcutaneous fat

Pyometra

Illustration 7.9   UROGENITAL SYSTEM

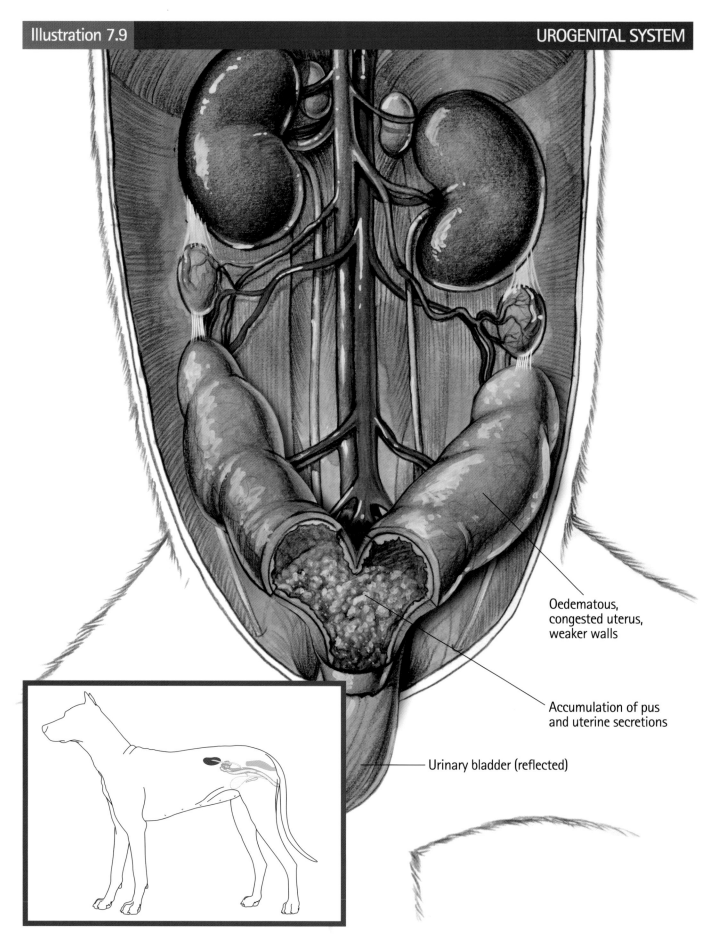

Oedematous, congested uterus, weaker walls

Accumulation of pus and uterine secretions

Urinary bladder (reflected)

Patent ductus arteriosus

Illustration 8.1   CARDIOVASCULAR SYSTEM

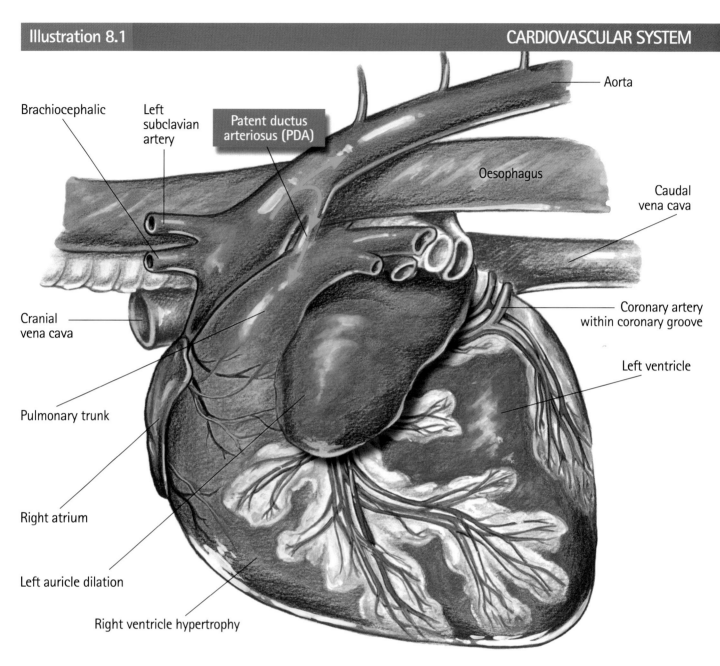

Aorta

Brachiocephalic

Left subclavian artery

Patent ductus arteriosus (PDA)

Oesophagus

Caudal vena cava

Cranial vena cava

Coronary artery within coronary groove

Left ventricle

Pulmonary trunk

Right atrium

Left auricle dilation

Right ventricle hypertrophy

BLOOD CIRCULATION DIAGRAM

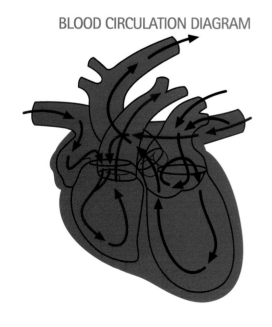

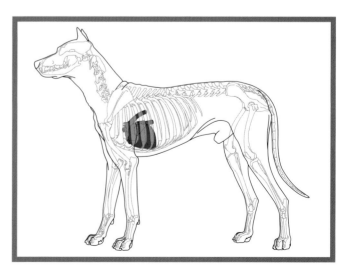

Pulmonary stenosis

Illustration 8.2 CARDIOVASCULAR SYSTEM

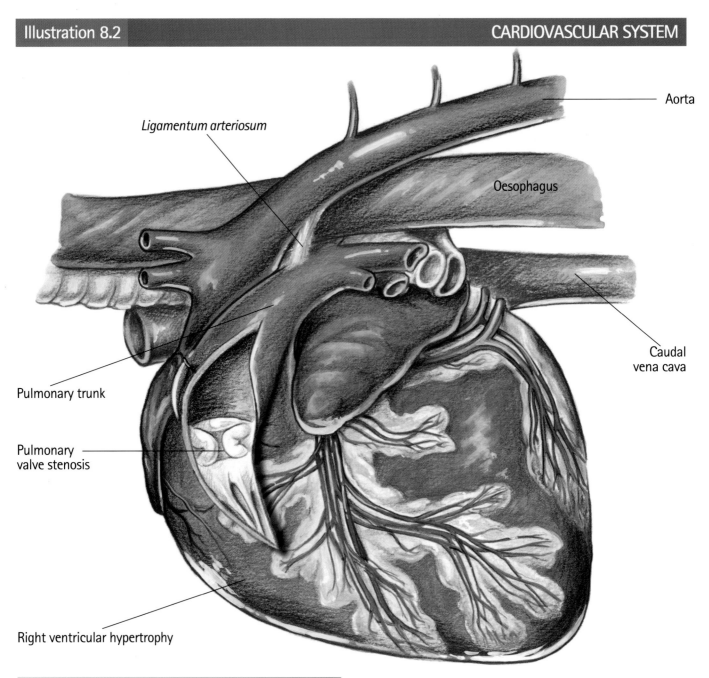

Ligamentum arteriosum

Aorta

Oesophagus

Caudal vena cava

Pulmonary trunk

Pulmonary valve stenosis

Right ventricular hypertrophy

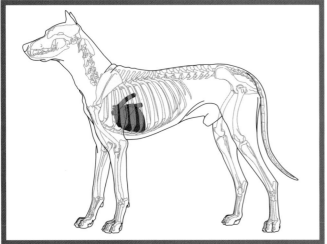

Aortic stenosis

Aorta

Oesophagus

Caudal vena cava

Left ventricle

Chordae tendineae

Right atrium

Aortic valve stenosis (valvular and subvalvular nodes)

Papillary muscles

Pulmonary valve

Right ventricle

Aortic semilunar valves

Ventricular septal defect

Illustration 8.4   CARDIOVASCULAR SYSTEM

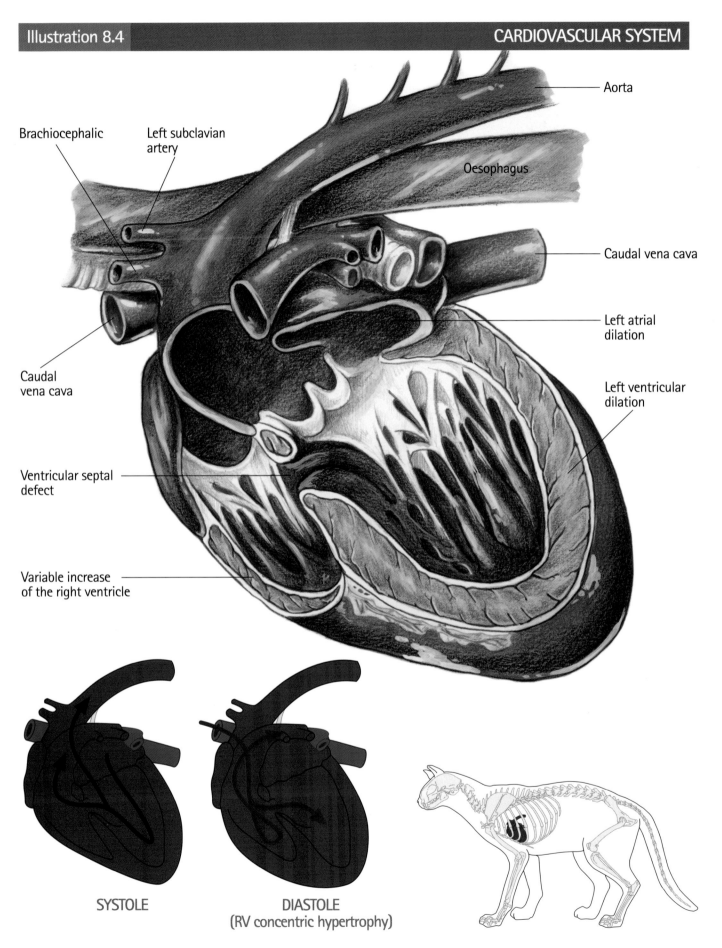

Aorta

Brachiocephalic

Left subclavian artery

Oesophagus

Caudal vena cava

Left atrial dilation

Caudal vena cava

Left ventricular dilation

Ventricular septal defect

Variable increase of the right ventricle

SYSTOLE

DIASTOLE
(RV concentric hypertrophy)

Tetralogy of Fallot

Illustration 8.5   CARDIOVASCULAR SYSTEM

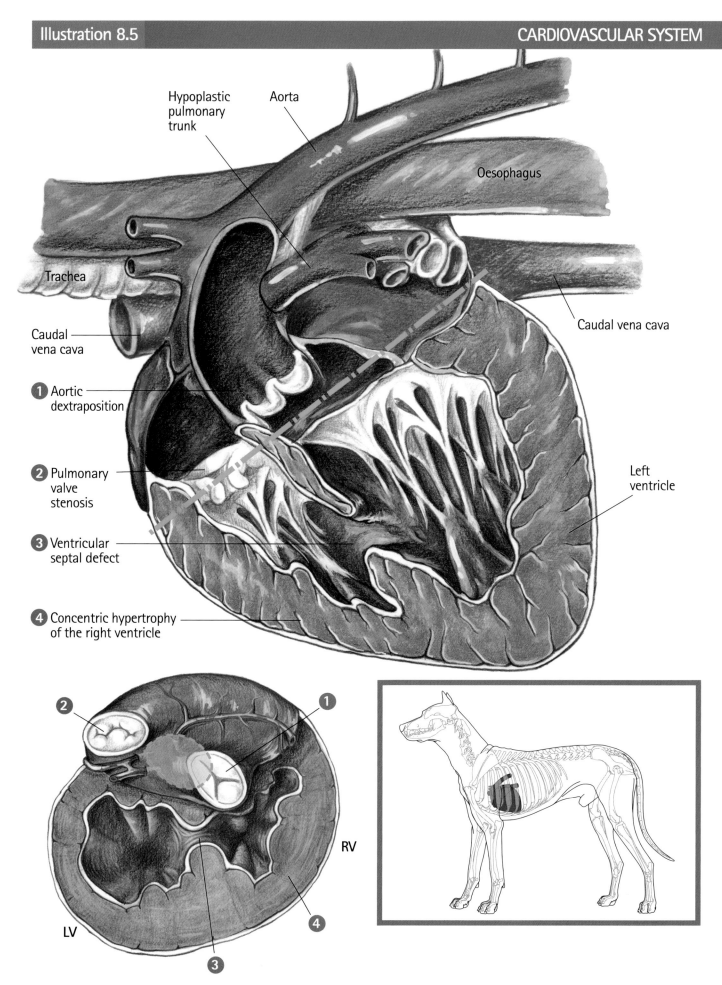

Hypoplastic pulmonary trunk

Aorta

Oesophagus

Trachea

Caudal vena cava

Caudal vena cava

1 Aortic dextraposition

2 Pulmonary valve stenosis

3 Ventricular septal defect

4 Concentric hypertrophy of the right ventricle

Left ventricle

RV

LV

Haemangiosarcoma/Pericardial effusion

Illustration 8.6   CARDIOVASCULAR SYSTEM

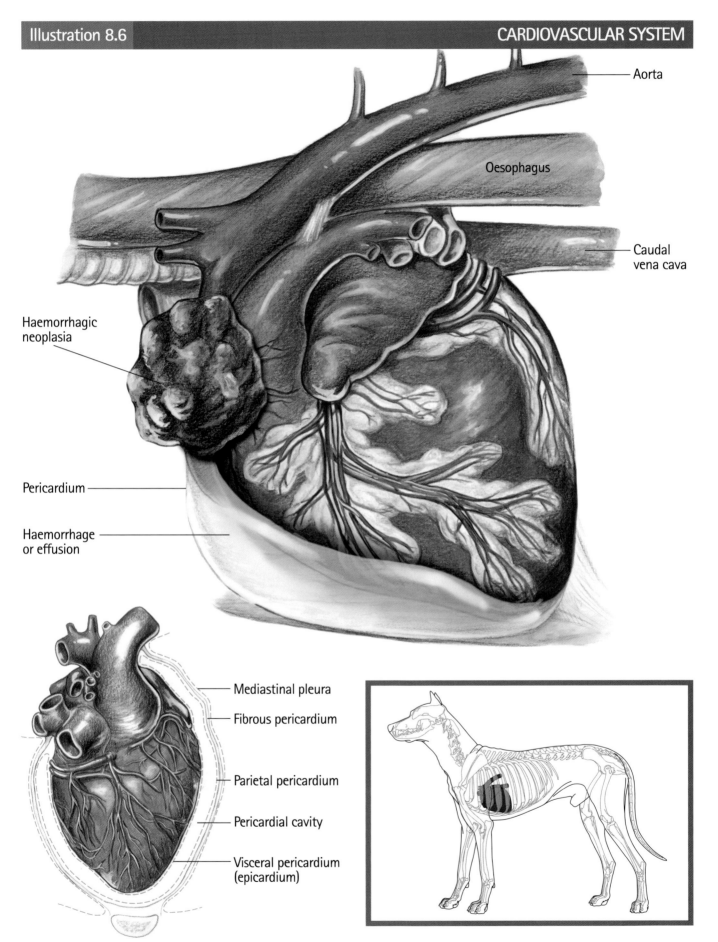

Aorta

Oesophagus

Caudal
vena cava

Haemorrhagic
neoplasia

Pericardium

Haemorrhage
or effusion

Mediastinal pleura

Fibrous pericardium

Parietal pericardium

Pericardial cavity

Visceral pericardium
(epicardium)

Tracheal collapse

Illustration 9.1   RESPIRATORY SYSTEM

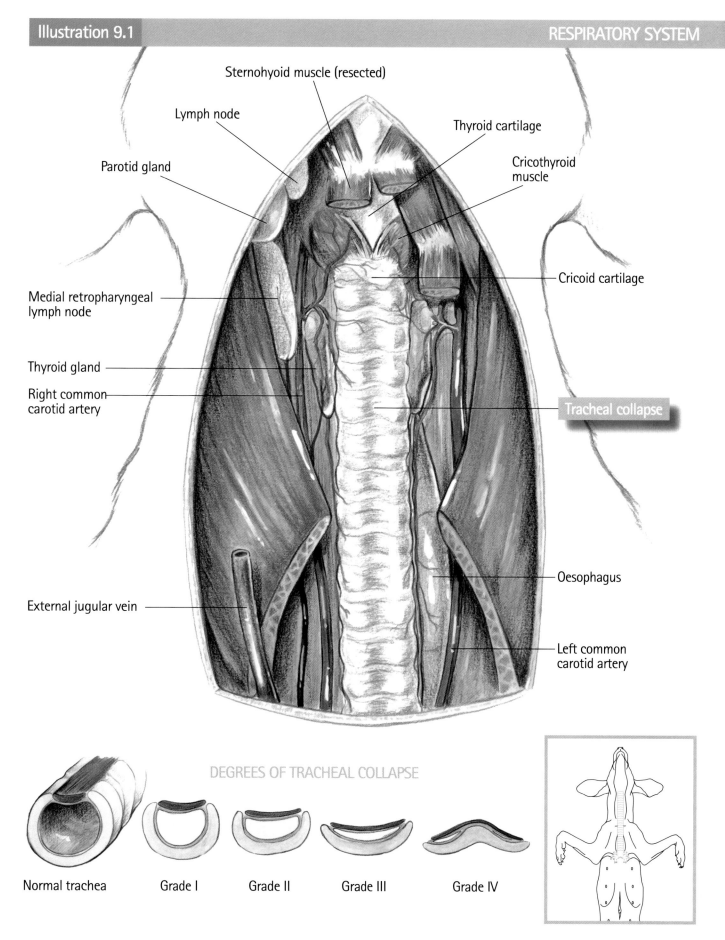

Sternohyoid muscle (resected)

Lymph node

Thyroid cartilage

Parotid gland

Cricothyroid muscle

Cricoid cartilage

Medial retropharyngeal lymph node

Thyroid gland

Right common carotid artery

Tracheal collapse

Oesophagus

External jugular vein

Left common carotid artery

DEGREES OF TRACHEAL COLLAPSE

Normal trachea   Grade I   Grade II   Grade III   Grade IV

Pulmonary neoplasia Partial lobectomy

Illustration 9.2 — RESPIRATORY SYSTEM

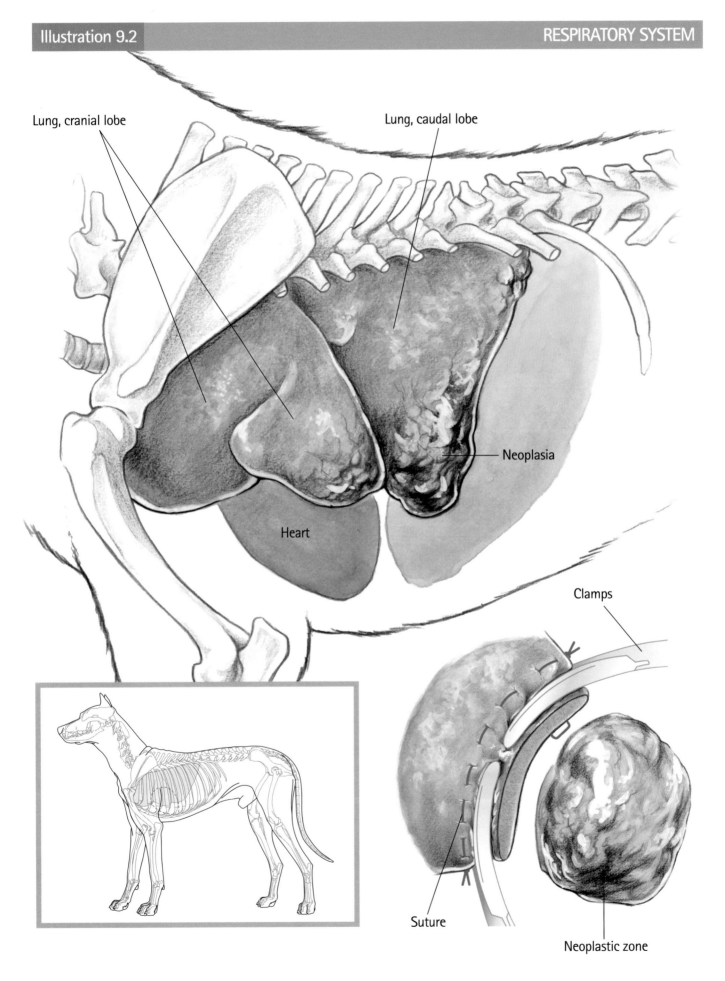

Lung, cranial lobe

Lung, caudal lobe

Neoplasia

Heart

Clamps

Suture

Neoplastic zone

Pleural effusion Drainage

Illustration 9.3

RESPIRATORY SYSTEM

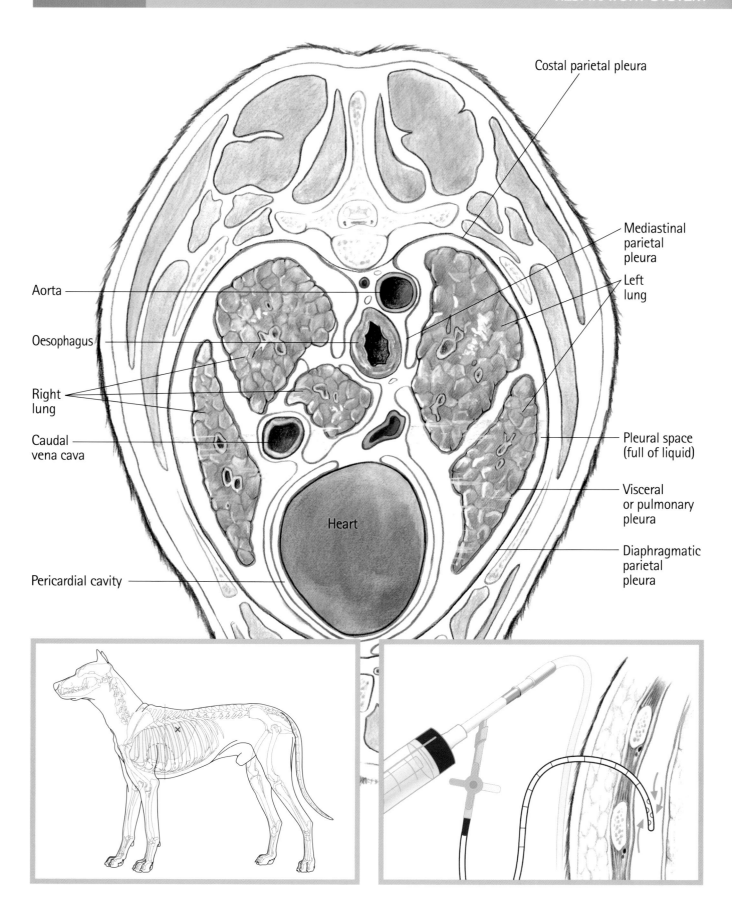

Costal parietal pleura

Mediastinal parietal pleura

Left lung

Aorta

Oesophagus

Right lung

Caudal vena cava

Pleural space (full of liquid)

Visceral or pulmonary pleura

Diaphragmatic parietal pleura

Heart

Pericardial cavity

Diaphragmatic hernia

Illustration 9.4   RESPIRATORY SYSTEM

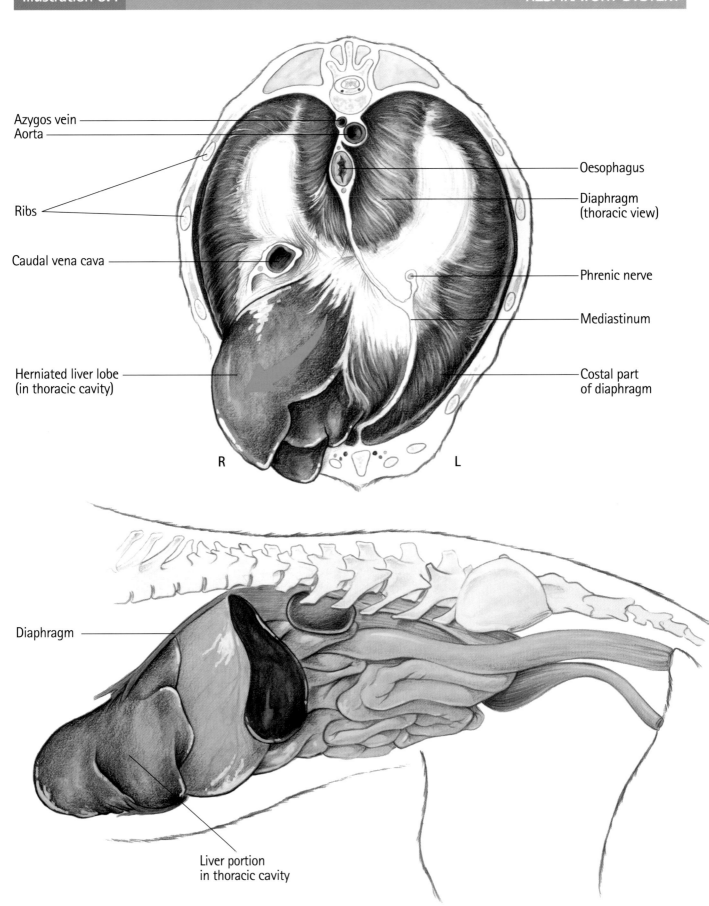

Azygos vein

Aorta

Oesophagus

Diaphragm
(thoracic view)

Ribs

Caudal vena cava

Phrenic nerve

Mediastinum

Herniated liver lobe
(in thoracic cavity)

Costal part
of diaphragm

R

L

Diaphragm

Liver portion
in thoracic cavity

Thymoma

Illustration 9.5   RESPIRATORY SYSTEM

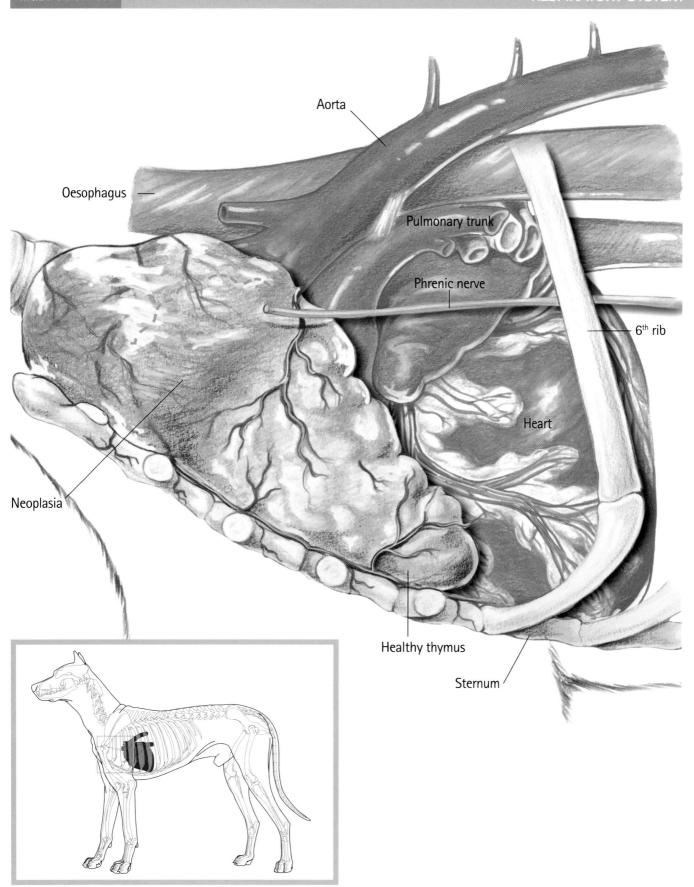

Aorta

Oesophagus

Pulmonary trunk

Phrenic nerve

6th rib

Heart

Neoplasia

Healthy thymus

Sternum

External fixator

Illustration 10.1   MUSCULOSKELETAL SYSTEM

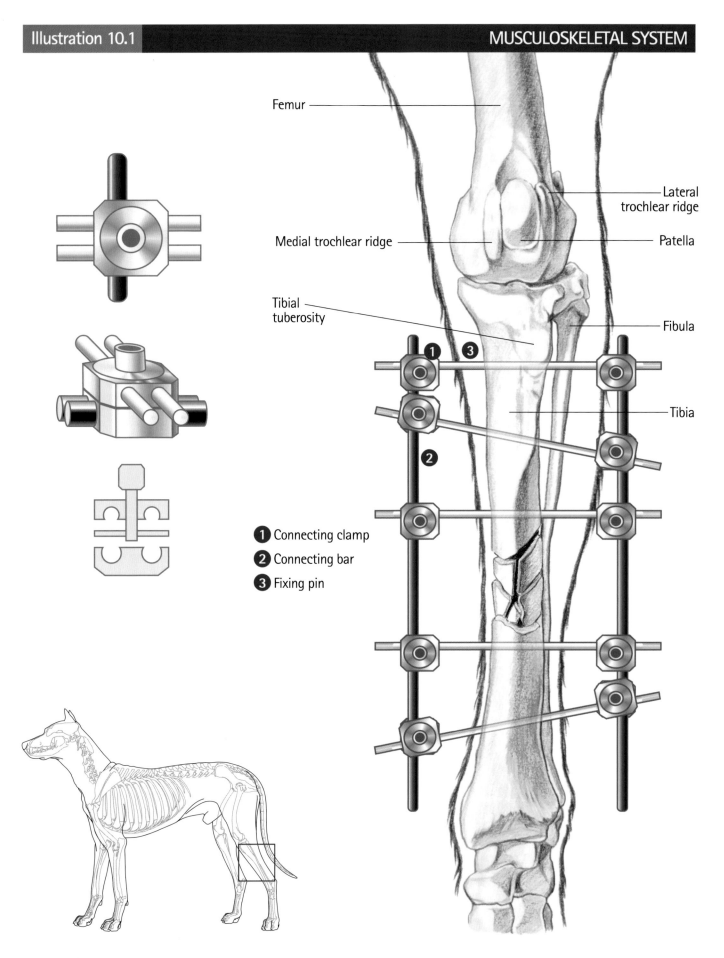

Femur

Lateral trochlear ridge

Medial trochlear ridge

Patella

Tibial tuberosity

Fibula

Tibia

1 Connecting clamp
2 Connecting bar
3 Fixing pin

Cerclage wire

Illustration 10.2   MUSCULOSKELETAL SYSTEM

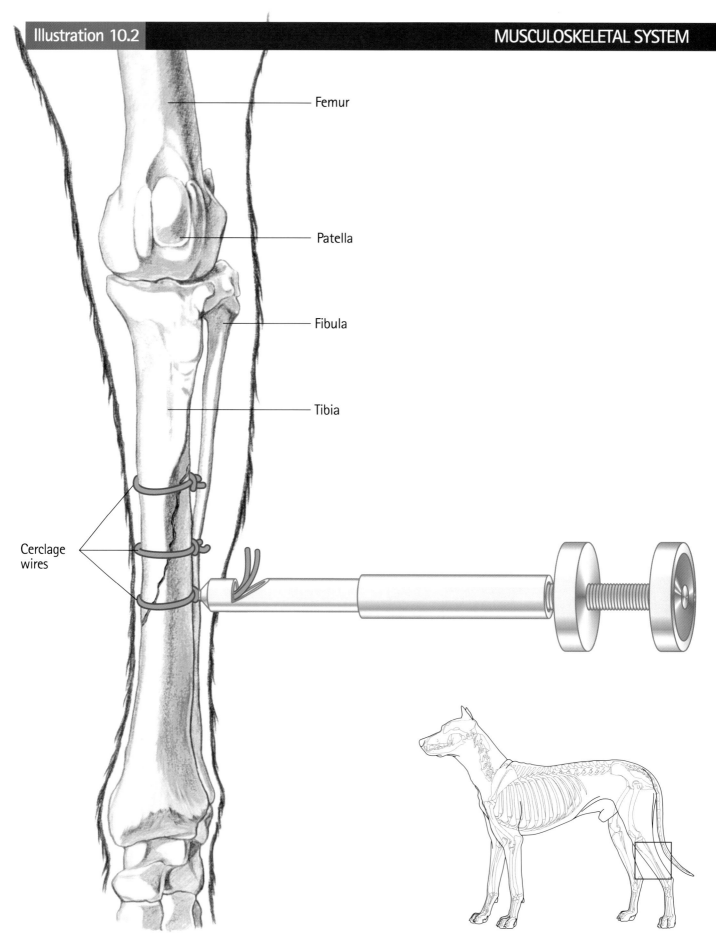

Femur

Patella

Fibula

Tibia

Cerclage
wires

Intramedullary pin

Illustration 10.3

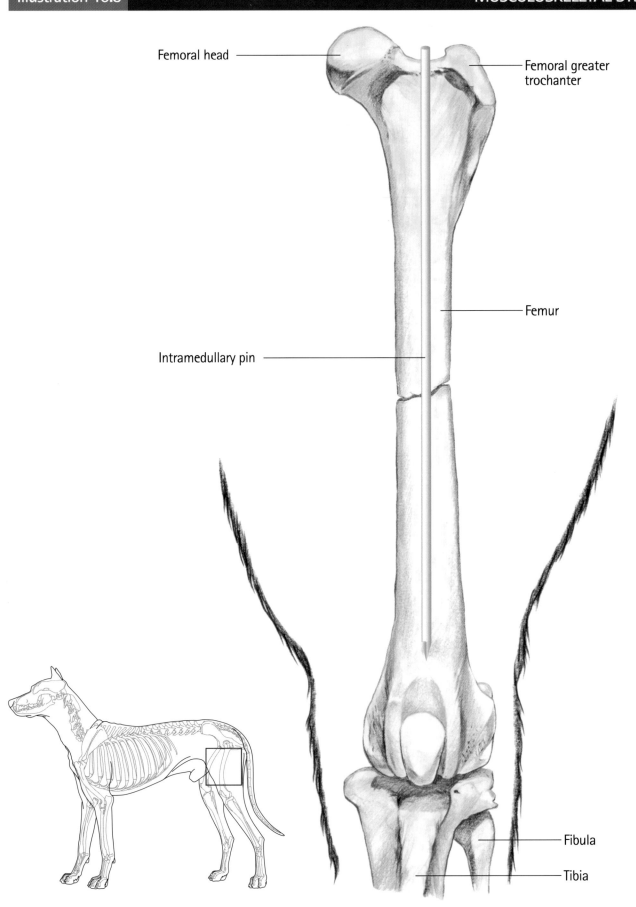

Femoral head

Femoral greater trochanter

Femur

Intramedullary pin

Fibula

Tibia

Tension band

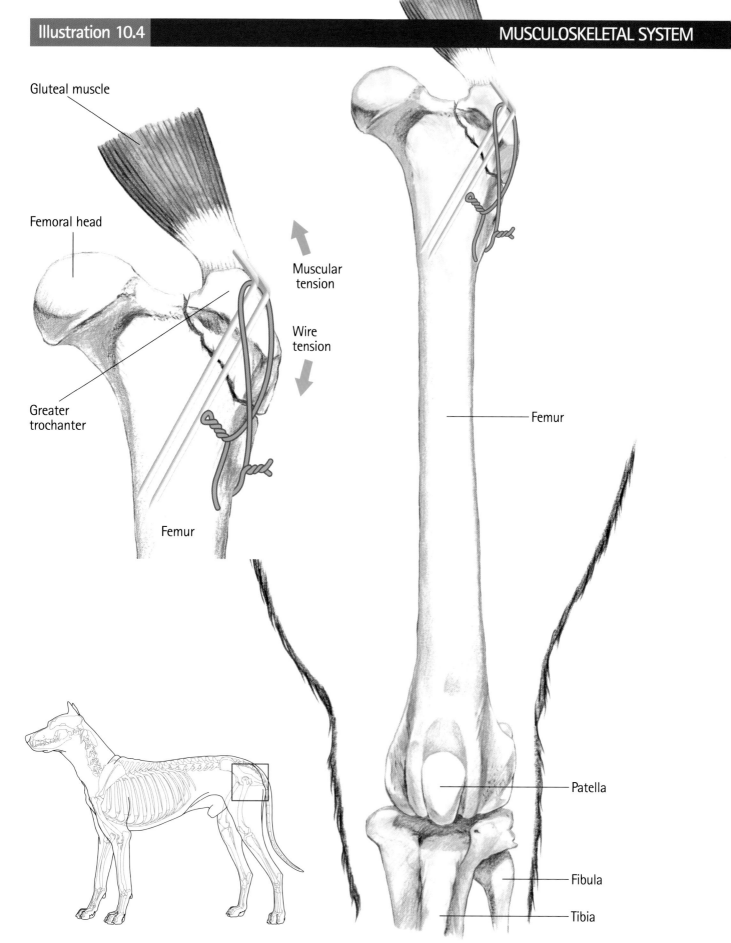

Gluteal muscle

Femoral head

Greater trochanter

Femur

Muscular tension

Wire tension

Femur

Patella

Fibula

Tibia

Internal fixation Screw + DCP plate

Illustration 10.5   MUSCULOSKELETAL SYSTEM

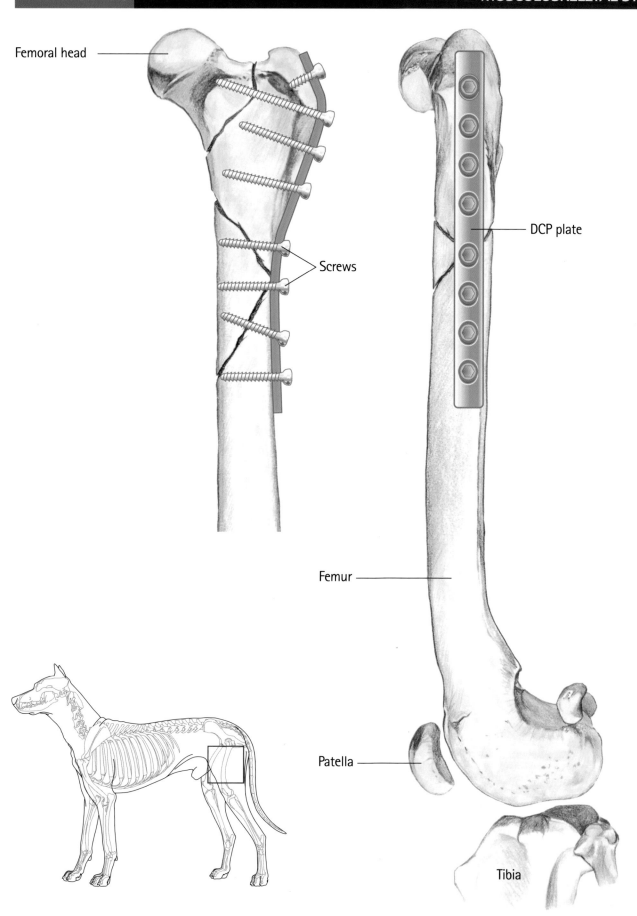

Femoral head

Screws

DCP plate

Femur

Patella

Tibia

Cranial cruciate ligament rupture

Illustration 10.6   MUSCULOSKELETAL SYSTEM

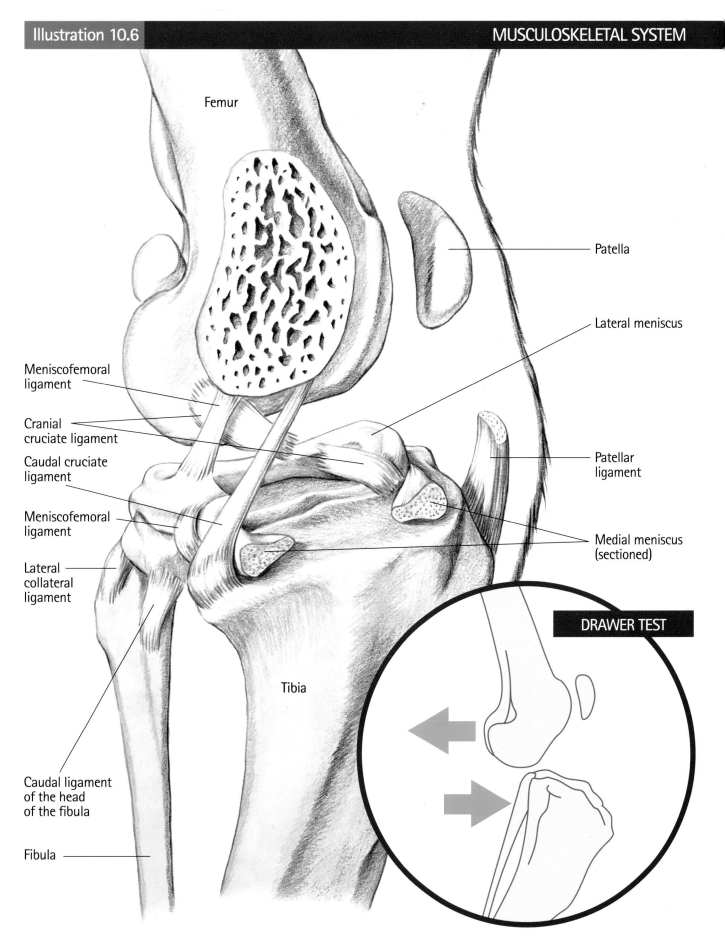

Femur

Patella

Lateral meniscus

Meniscofemoral ligament

Cranial cruciate ligament

Patellar ligament

Caudal cruciate ligament

Meniscofemoral ligament

Medial meniscus (sectioned)

Lateral collateral ligament

Tibia

DRAWER TEST

Caudal ligament of the head of the fibula

Fibula

TPLO (Tibial plateau levelling osteotomy)

Illustration 10.7

MUSCULOSKELETAL SYSTEM

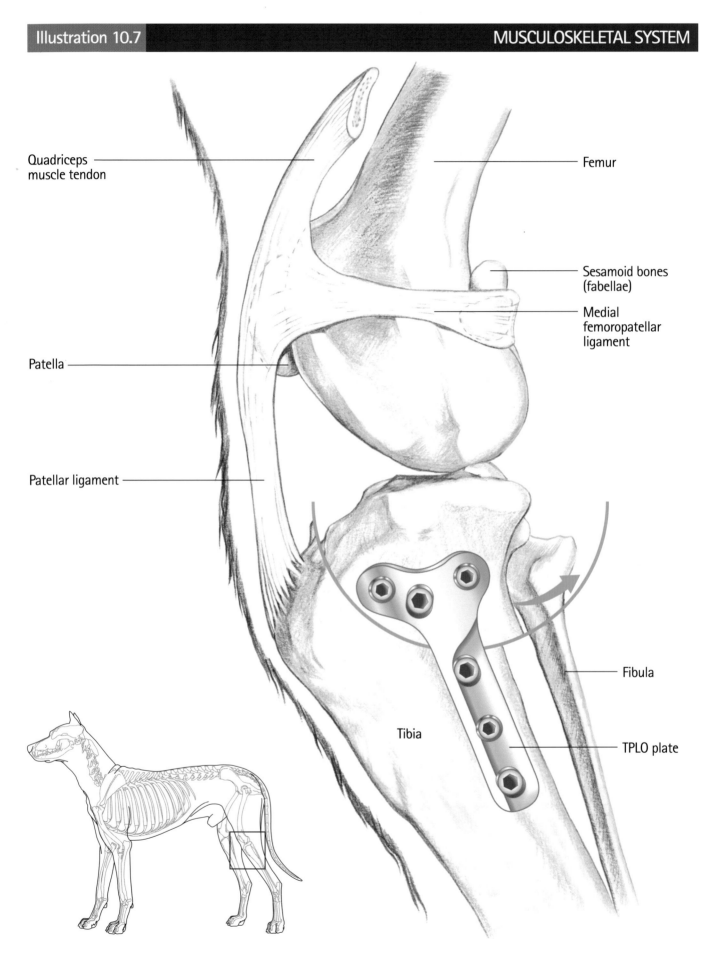

Quadriceps
muscle tendon

Femur

Sesamoid bones
(fabellae)

Medial
femoropatellar
ligament

Patella

Patellar ligament

Fibula

Tibia

TPLO plate

TTA (Tibial tuberosity advancement)

Illustration 10.8   MUSCULOSKELETAL SYSTEM

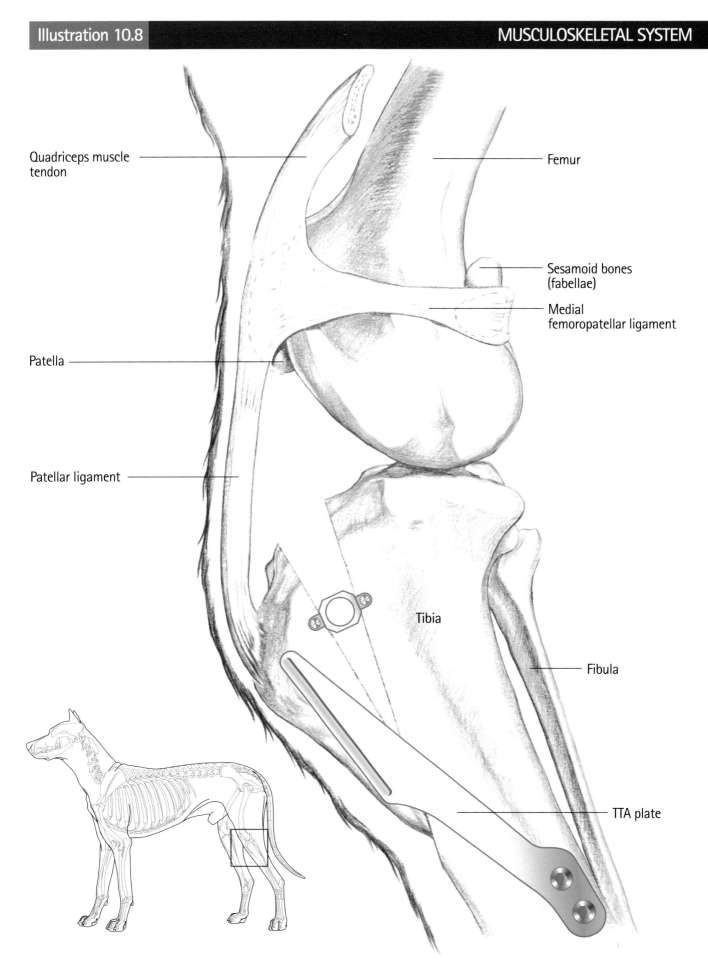

Quadriceps muscle tendon

Femur

Sesamoid bones (fabellae)

Medial femoropatellar ligament

Patella

Patellar ligament

Tibia

Fibula

TTA plate

Wedge osteotomy

Illustration 10.9   MUSCULOSKELETAL SYSTEM

Quadriceps muscle tendon

Femur

Sesamoids (fabellae)

Patella

Medial femoropatellar ligament

Patellar ligament

Tibia

Fibula

Fabellotibial suture

Illustration 10.10

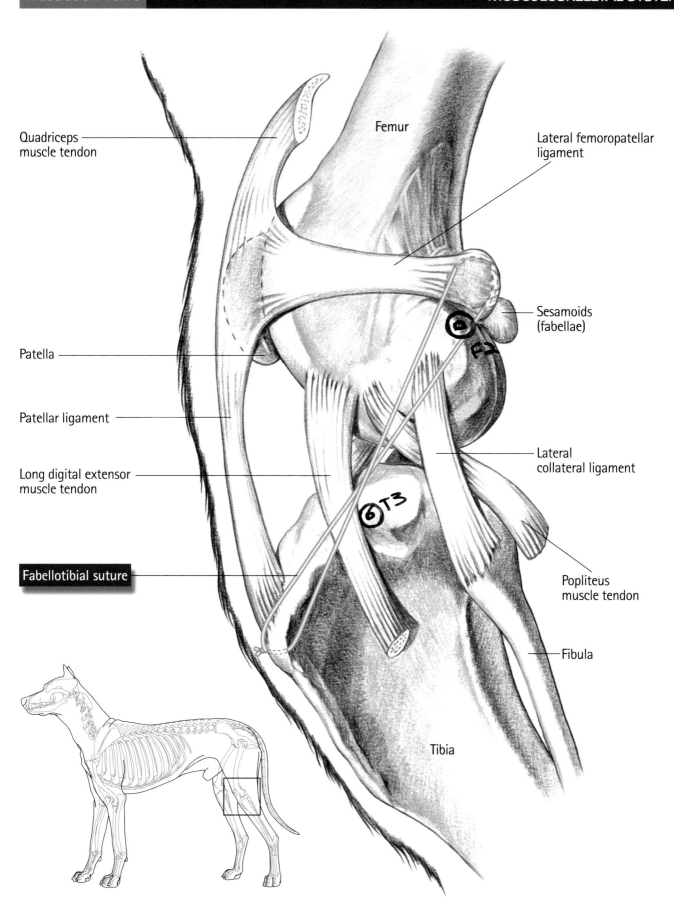

Quadriceps
muscle tendon

Femur

Lateral femoropatellar
ligament

Sesamoids
(fabellae)

Patella

Patellar ligament

Long digital extensor
muscle tendon

Lateral
collateral ligament

Fabellotibial suture

Popliteus
muscle tendon

Fibula

Tibia

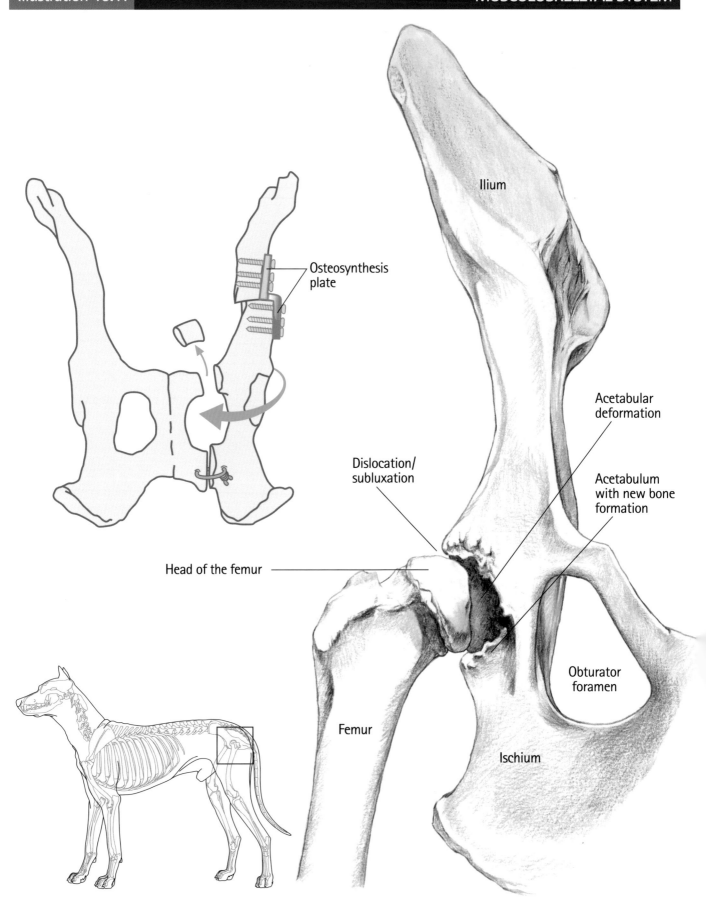

Osteosynthesis plate

Head of the femur

Ilium

Acetabular deformation

Acetabulum with new bone formation

Dislocation/ subluxation

Obturator foramen

Femur

Ischium

Shoulder OCD (Osteochondritis dissecans)

Illustration 10.12   MUSCULOSKELETAL SYSTEM

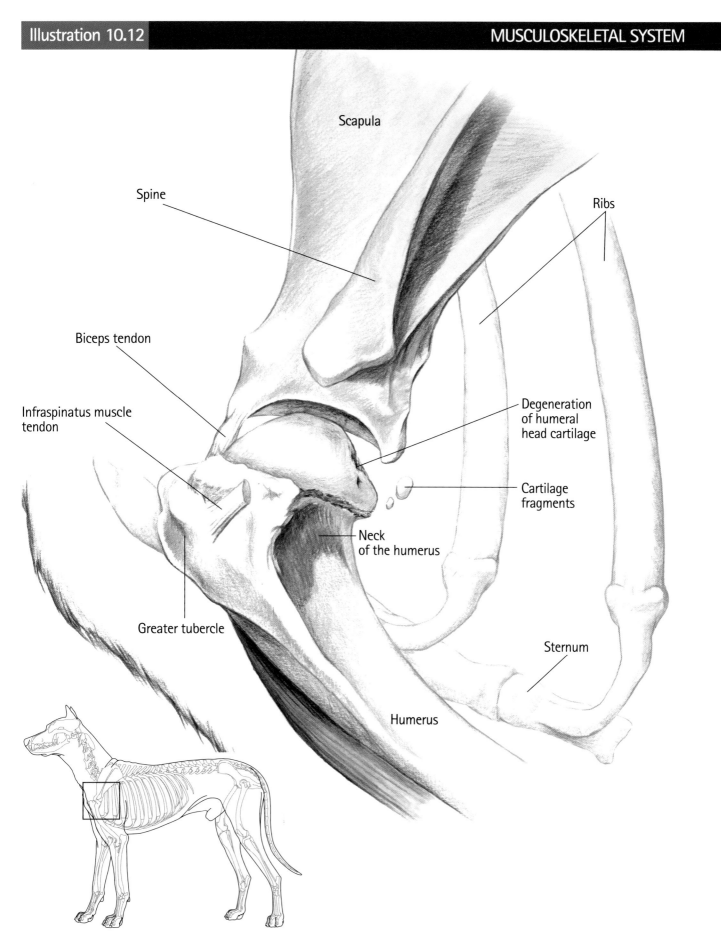

Scapula

Spine

Ribs

Biceps tendon

Infraspinatus muscle tendon

Degeneration of humeral head cartilage

Cartilage fragments

Neck of the humerus

Greater tubercle

Sternum

Humerus

Intervertebral disc extrusion: Laminectomy

Illustration 10.13   MUSCULOSKELETAL SYSTEM

Spinous process

Mammillary process

Spinal cord

Vertebral venous siuses

Ventral longitudinal ligament

Fibrous ring

Herniated nucleus pulposus

Spinal nerves

Transverse process

Intervertebral disc

Hernia

Ununited anconeal process Elbow dysplasia

Illustration 10.14   MUSCULOSKELETAL SYSTEM

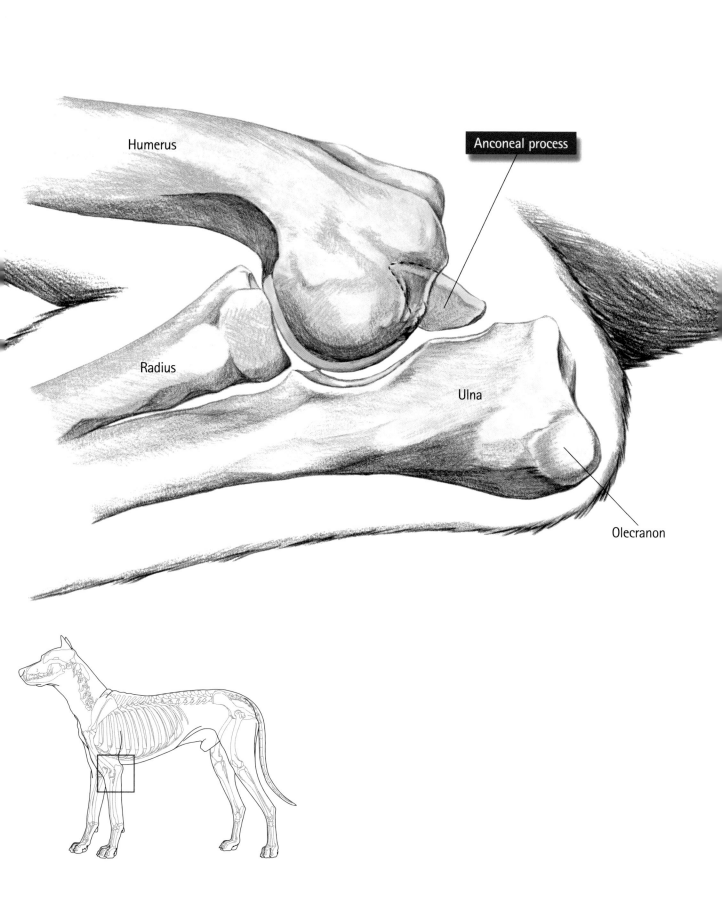

Humerus

Anconeal process

Radius

Ulna

Olecranon

Fragmented medial coronoid process

Illustration 10.15   MUSCULOSKELETAL SYSTEM

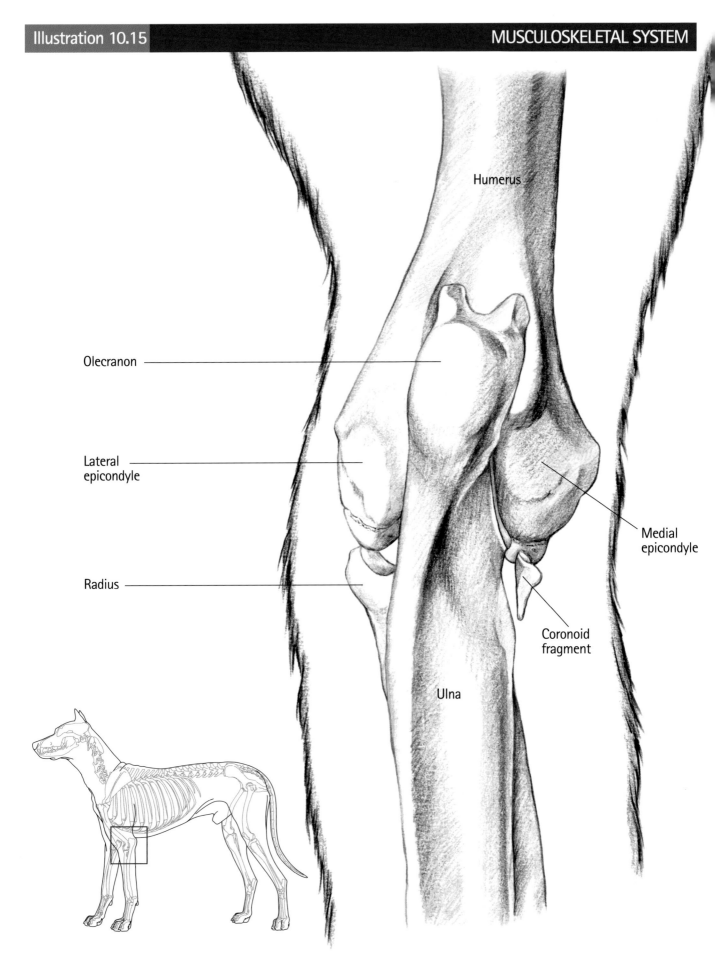

Humerus

Olecranon

Lateral
epicondyle

Radius

Medial
epicondyle

Coronoid
fragment

Ulna

Stifle arthroscopy

Illustration 10.16

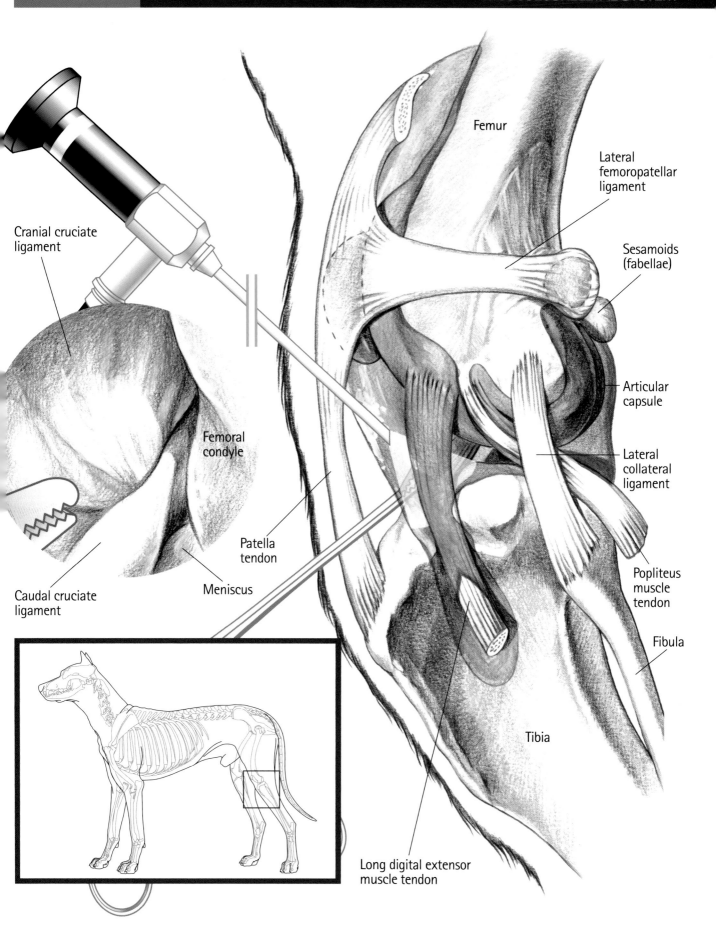

Cranial cruciate ligament

Femoral condyle

Caudal cruciate ligament

Meniscus

Patella tendon

Femur

Lateral femoropatellar ligament

Sesamoids (fabellae)

Articular capsule

Lateral collateral ligament

Popliteus muscle tendon

Fibula

Tibia

Long digital extensor muscle tendon

Total hip replacement

Illustration 10.17

Ilium

Femoral head and neck

Reconstructed acetabulum

Total hip replacement

Ischium

Meniscal injury

Illustration 10.18   MUSCULOSKELETAL SYSTEM

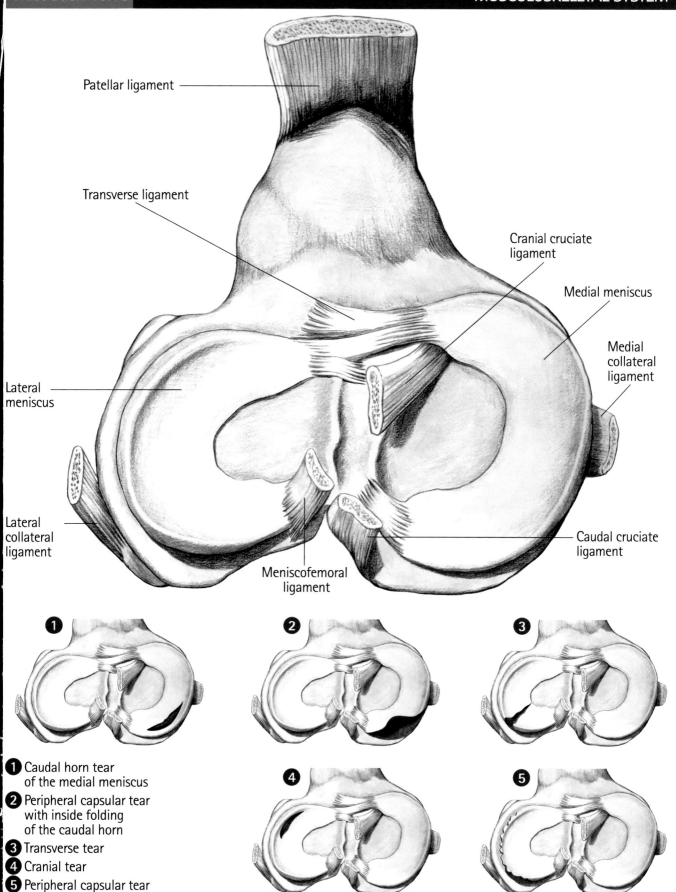

Patellar ligament

Transverse ligament

Cranial cruciate ligament

Medial meniscus

Medial collateral ligament

Lateral meniscus

Lateral collateral ligament

Meniscofemoral ligament

Caudal cruciate ligament

❶ Caudal horn tear of the medial meniscus
❷ Peripheral capsular tear with inside folding of the caudal horn
❸ Transverse tear
❹ Cranial tear
❺ Peripheral capsular tear

Patellar luxation

Illustration 10.19   MUSCULOSKELETAL SYSTEM

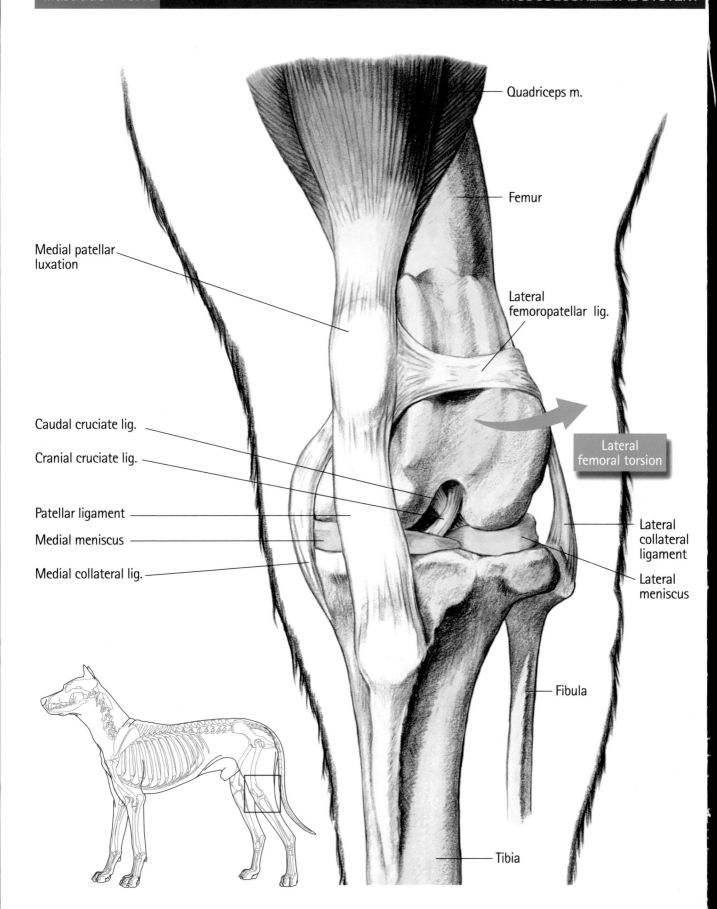

Quadriceps m.

Femur

Medial patellar luxation

Lateral femoropatellar lig.

Caudal cruciate lig.

Cranial cruciate lig.

Lateral femoral torsion

Patellar ligament

Medial meniscus

Medial collateral lig.

Lateral collateral ligament

Lateral meniscus

Fibula

Tibia